THE POWER OF PERSONAL HEALTH

Jack Schwarz, a pioneer in the education health field, has gained worldwide recognition for his work. He is the president of the Aletheia Foundation, which he founded in 1958, and has been a subject, researcher, and consultant at major bio-medical and life science research centers in the United States and abroad. Results of tests performed on Jack document his abilities to self-regulate many psycho-physiological processes.

The Power of Personal Health is the latest in a series of books in which Jack Schwarz explores the dynamics of health education, always with an emphasis on energy and self-regulation. He is dedicated to educating others in self-health and awareness, and bringing together research on health and human energies.

For further information on Jack Schwarz and the Aletheia Foundation, contact: Aletheia Foundation, 515 N.E. 8th Street, Grants Pass, OR 97526; (503) 479–4855.

THE POWER OF PERSONAL HEALTH

JACK SCHWARZ

ARKANA

ARKANA
Published by the Penguin Group
Viking Penguin, a division of Penguin Books USA Inc.,
375 Hudson Street, New York, New York 10014, U.S.A.
Penguin Books Ltd, 27 Wrights Lane,
London W8 5TZ, England
Penguin Books Australia Ltd, Ringwood,
Victoria, Australia
Penguin Books Canada Ltd, 10 Alcorn Avenue, Suite 300,
Toronto, Ontario, Canada M4V, 3B2
Penguin Books (N.Z.) Ltd, 182–190 Wairau Road,
Auckland 10, New Zealand

Penguin Books Ltd, Registered Offices:
Harmondsworth, Middlesex, England

First published in Arkana Books 1992

1 3 5 7 9 10 8 6 4 2

LIBRARY OF CONGRESS CATALOGING IN PUBLICATION DATA
Schwarz, Jack, 1924–
The power of personal health / Jack Schwarz.
p.   cm.
ISBN 0 14 019.453 3
1. Health.   2. Natural immunity—Psychological aspects.   3. Mind
and body.   I. Title.
RA776.S385   1992
613—dc20   91–42242

Printed in the United States of America
Set in Weiss
Designed by Brian Mulligan

To all those searching
for their own truth
and better health.

Thank you to all
involved in making
this book possible.

—Jack Schwarz

PREFACE: PROGRESSIVE EXCITEMENT

Health is not a constant state, but a dynamic evolutionary process in which one second is never the same as the other.

Excitement is a state of high energy in which body, mind, and spirit act as a whole, radiating without the need for self-protection. Keeping a high level of energy involves continually changing and adapting to the world, being in a state of progressive excitement. I never oppose life's continuous changes, and therefore I never stagnate.

While many may think that it takes a lot of energy to change, the truth is that energy is continually and naturally changing and our task is to live in rhythm with these natural changes. All disease is caused by fear of change! When we fear change, we withdraw and stagnate and thus have low resistance. If we do not fear change, we can respond spontaneously to life.

We all need to learn to value excitement and to understand how it helps us flow with changes and open up to our own inner being. Then we will be able to begin our self-healing and realize our true potentials.

Stay excited! That is the way to health, peace, and love.

CONTENTS

THE POWER OF PERSONAL HEALTH

1

THE
IMMUNE SYSTEM
OF THE WORLD

Great changes are taking place today—political, social, technological, and particularly changes in our levels of consciousness. I know you are concerned with these changes, not only in your own life, but in the lives of everyone throughout the world. That is why we need to consider how our consciousness relates to what I call the "immune system of the world." This is the physical and spiritual energy on our planet that protects the health of our environment, our societies, and every individual.

Just as the body's immune system can become deficient,

so can the world immune system fail. Today, in the 1990s, the cause of the world's immune deficiency is the illness of our politics, our intolerance for individual and cultural differences, and ignorance of our own inner lives.

Modern science has learned a great deal about the physiology of the body's immune system, although even today we cannot find the thymus gland or the pineal gland on most anatomical charts. You may have heard that the thymus gland atrophies after the age of thirteen—as if when God created the human body, He thought, "Well, let me put in a thymus gland, even though they won't need it. And I'll hang that useless pineal gland between the two hemispheres of the brain and maybe some people will call it the Third Eye." Scientists used to think the appendix was useless, too. Several million were taken out because we thought it was a vestigial organ, only there to become infected. Eventually we discovered that the appendix plays an important role in intestinal tract metabolism and enzyme production.

It is now clear to researchers that all glands are interdependent and necessary for the functioning of the immune system. The human body may appear to be solid, but it is a complex energy system, and we cannot treat each part separately and ignore the rest. It is particularly significant that we often overlook the thymus. Metaphysically, the thymus gland is the heart center, the heart chakra. It is that part of our being that works with the various levels of consciousness and transmutes energy from solidity to the more refined energy of our higher nature, which is one with the nature of the universe.

In my opinion, the United States is the heart center of the world, the thymus of the world immune system. I came to the United States about thirty years ago and like many others I did not know at the time exactly why I came. Now I see that this is the new Holy Land, the heart center where consciousness needs to be awakened and then networked out all over the world. But the United States does not always provide the right kind of leadership, and the world immune system is faltering. To restore the health of our world, all of us here in the United States must begin to play the part of the thymus and transform our consciousness to a higher level.

For many people, the first step must be to recognize consciousness as the great mover and shaker in the world. For example, when I was still a boy, I learned from my own experience that the mind could control bleeding and pain. Later, under laboratory conditions, I demonstrated that ability by putting a long sail maker's needle through my body. I had no pain or physiological trauma, and when the needle was pulled out there was no bleeding. The wounds healed immediately, even when the needles were contaminated with viruses, bacteria, or infected tissue. Not once in thirty-three years of these experiments did an infection occur. I was studied extensively, but for many years my ability was considered only an amazing physical feat. It was some time before scientists in the United States began to understand that I was demonstrating voluntary autogenic control of my immune system—a feat of consciousness.

One reason more of us have not developed this ability is that the thinking process taught in the Western world emphasizes doubt and questioning at the expense of spontaneity and inner knowing. We learn to be suspicious of taking action unless we think we know the outcome in advance. We hold back, fearful of unpremeditated action. Then the flow of our being becomes inhibited, and the stagnated energy interferes with the healthy functioning of the body's immune system.

A physician might tell you that you caught a cold because "your resistance was low." That also means you have a low voltage and low output. You are holding on to your energy because you don't know what will happen next. Imagine if the sun acted that way! The sun doesn't know what happens when it shines. Why should you? So let your energy radiate. You will make a lot of people happy with your sunshine, and you will have a high resistance level. Any scientist will tell you that it is impossible to introduce a lower energy field into a higher energy field. Maintain a high enough energy field around you, and no disease will be able to affect you.

Our Western bias against spontaneous activity prevents us from recognizing how the mind can naturally direct the body. Many scientists still believe that the mind is no more than the thinking process taking place in the brain. But we know that the brain is like a computer; it is only an instrument used by the mind to program and operate the body. The mind is the directing part of our being, the source of energy from which all of us are created. The mind is not a separate part of the world, not an invisible plastic bubble in which we walk around, but an indivisible aspect of the energy of the entire universe. This energy cannot be created or destroyed; it can only be transformed. The mind directs the transformation of energy in a natural, dynamic evolutionary process. If we allow our consciousness to flow with that process, the body's immune system can respond spontaneously to the energy transformations taking place around us.

Health is maintained by partaking of those transformations—willingly, consciously, decisively—whether they are cosmic changes on the scale of the universe, movements in world events, or physical and emotional activities in our bodies. The more each of us can become aware of the levels of consciousness that regulate the immune system, the healthier we can be, and the healthier our world can become. This is especially true for us here in the United States, where we are taught that health is a static balance, which must be defended against disease with prescription drugs and surgery.

There is a basic law of energy transformation, stated by Einstein, that may help us gain a new perspective on health, consciousness, and the state of our world. The law is: *the more momentum radiant energy has, the more time slows down;* and conversely, the less momentum, or more inertia, energy has, the more time speeds up. In physics, this law applies to the behavior of the particles that make up the universe. In our own lives, we can see this law at work in the way our personal energy either maintains our youthful vigor or allows our health to deteriorate and our bodies to age prematurely.

Look at people who are depressed, repressed, and suppressed. Their hesitation to act with spontaneity and a high level of consciousness creates inertia, which causes energy to stagnate in their bodies. Their energy loses momentum and their immune systems become deficient. They become diseased, weak, and old before their time.

Look at people who challenge life without inhibition and self-doubt. Their energy flows and radiates, maintaining its momentum, and their immune systems are intact. The result is an extended healthy life. It would not be strange for us to to be able to live to 150 and still be active.

We must remember that our bodies are only intermediate stages in the natural transformations of radiant energy. This energy begins as electro-potential. It condenses under the influence of gravity into the more rigid forms of molecular chemistry. Then it expands and flows again, and finally radiates out into the universe. Each of us has the potential to become aware of this cycle in our own lives. We can learn to use our consciousness to activate our energy whenever it becomes stagnated in the biochemistry of the physical body. The power and radiance of our inner energy when it expands is what protects our bodies from infection and disease. That is what we call the immune system. And the more all of us release our energies and become radiant, the stronger the world immune system will become. Then the world can become a healthier environment, a place where we can face life as a creative challenge and live every day with excitement and love.

I know people who say we can help others who have stagnated, and whose immune systems are depleted, by sending them light. By this they mean allowing what we call the transpersonal self, the higher self, or the divine self, to resonate with radiant energy from a higher level, activating our whole being—physiologically, emotionally, mentally, and spiritually.

When people are healthy and radiant, they send out and receive energy in the form of light. This radiance can, in fact, activate the immune system. But in my experience, most people, even with the best of intentions, are probably not sending out light, because they really do not know how to be radiant.

The task facing us is to learn how to be an instrument to help others go beyond inertia, to show others that we do not have to be controlled by our environment—by conformity, pollution, war, consumerism, or despair. Instead, we can control our environment and our own lives. But we must begin by recognizing how much we need to learn.

Here in America we have a society and a history rich in opportunities to transmute consciousness to a higher level. We can begin by examining the attitudes that create inertia and lead to destructiveness and disease. The expansion of the Western frontier and the fate of Native American peoples is one of our most important lessons. We fought wars of extermination against the American Indians. Then we tried to assimilate them into our culture. We wanted them to cut their hair, adopt our dress and language, and wear shoes instead of walking on bare feet. And, of course, we tried to force them to adapt to our Western diet. But they could not adapt to a way of life so out of tune with nature and spirit. The legacy of the frontier has been a century of deceit, repression, and guilt—

all of which weaken the immune system and contribute to the emotional and health problems of the present.

What we need to do, as individuals and as a whole, is recognize that there is a great need for love—unconditional love. To me, the word "love" represents:

L – Life
O – Omnipresent
V – Victoriously
E – Expressed

By "life omnipresent" I mean that life is present in all things. It is not only in human beings, but in animals, trees, rocks—in every living thing, every object. Even a table is composed of the same energy as we are. It is part of the interrelated whole. It has its function and is going through its own transformational process. The same is true of the 75 trillion cells that make up the human body, and of every particle in each of those cells. Not a single one is exactly like another, and each has its own destiny. If we can accept this truth, perhaps we can learn to stop judging other things and other beings by limited human or cultural standards. That would be a great advance, for it is judging that holds us back from giving and receiving unconditional love.

By "victoriously expressed" I mean getting joy and love out of life every day. We can accept change as an exciting challenge and use our energy to expand and become radiant. We do not need to live in a state of fear and anxiety. It is no good to be obsessed with defending ourselves against enemies and fighting disease. Instead, we can encircle ourselves with expanding energy. Then we can resonate with each other in a natural healthy state of spiritual power.

American society, for all of its freedom, too often imposes average standards on us. We are encouraged to judge anyone or anything that differs too much from the norm as a threat to our health and way of life. No matter how strong our institutions, we feel surrounded by dangers against which we must mobilize our whole defense system. We would do better if we could resist labeling so many things as enemies. If we could see "threats" as challenges to stimulate our inner potential, we could start radiating light that would really protect us. We don't realize that "defense" actually opens the gates for everything we don't want to get into our energy. When we think we are defending ourselves, we have leaking, sievelike energy fields around us, and depressed immune systems.

A healthy society should be composed of radiant individuals who are not offended by differences and do not need to live in a continual state of defense. In such a society, we would not judge others. Instead, we would discern within ourselves what is appropriate and what is inappropriate for our own growth. We would accept that no two of us are the same and enjoy that diversity.

All too often, we are fearful because we are ignorant of our own inner selves. And if we cannot understand ourselves, how can we expect to understand and unconditionally love those around us? Or the people down the block? Or in the next city or the next country? Or people of different races or religions?

Many of us in the United States believe we are healing-oriented, but we still give power to disease by focusing on specific symptoms. Let me give you an analogy. We will think of America as a body, and El Salvador a tumor in that body. If America sends all of its troops to conquer the tumor, what happens to America's immune system? It becomes absolutely depleted. We may be victorious in defeating El Salvador, but the rest of the body falls apart because there is no defense system left.

We see this happen with people who are victorious over a specific disease, absolutely free of it. Then, a few months later, they die of seemingly natural causes. An autopsy shows no sign of the original disease. Often, from a scientific point of view, we do not know what caused death. I say, however, that the immune system was used up fighting the one specific disease in one specific part of the body.

It is the same when someone asks me to help heal

a specific medical problem: "Jack, I have a brother, Robert Jones, with a kidney problem. He lives at 1450 Oak Street, Apt. 45, New York City. We want to avoid an operation if at all possible, so would you please send him some absent healing for his kidneys?"

First of all, I do not want to know his name or where he lives or what his disease is. I do not want to pay attention to the symptoms instead of the whole. Besides, if I were to go to work and visualize his kidney, and even if I were to claim that it is the power of God working through me, do I doubt that God knows His way around the universe? Do I have to tell Him who and where it is? Do I need to draw Him a map?

Assuming that I could heal the kidneys, wouldn't I thereby deny the rest of Mr. Jones? Isn't his little toe as diseased as his kidneys? Although his toe may show no symptoms, it cannot function the way it could because the kidneys are not functioning as they should. Mr. Jones is not just a kidney or a little toe, but a whole being who needs to be brought back to perfection of soul, mind, and body.

Until we overcome our inertia and treat the whole, our diets and remedies and cures will not be effective. Someone once commented that American urine is the most expensive in the world. It is loaded with vitamins and minerals that our bodies cannot assimilate, because our energy is stagnated. And, as I observe the energy that flows from most of us, it looks like molasses. The mass is so thick! Our thoughts are fearful, always wondering what will happen to us next. There is no self-knowingness that nothing can happen to us unless we let it happen.

I traveled to China in 1981. Before I had this opportunity to be with the Chinese people, I had been influenced by the Western opinion that the Chinese were stoic, that they didn't show or express their emotions. However, I found the Chinese to have an energy that was very much a contained state of excitement that could simply be felt when you came into their presence.

Here in the West, we have a lot of hip-hip-hurrah energy. We are all excitable: "Oh, wow, it's great to see you here! Isn't that fantastic!" But underneath our excitability is a fearfulness of ulterior motives: "What's he doing? Why is he picking me out of all these people? Either I'm special or there's something wrong with me."

If you want your thymus gland and your immune system to function effectively, start looking at the judgments you make about yourself and others that may be stagnating your flow of energy. To prevent disease, we must prevent inertia within ourselves. Then we can be instrumental in helping others overcome inertia by sharing our beingness, by giving off the higher power that comes from our body, mind, and soul's being in total harmony.

Recognize that you do not need to back away from people who are different from you. Open your arms to new experiences because if you keep yourself running on a high energy level, nothing negative can affect you. I know that if I let down my energy and allow myself to get aggravated by what someone says or does, I may soon have a sniffle or a cold.

Once I was invited to see a man who had served as a missionary in a foreign country. He had tried to bring another race to God by convincing them to give up what he considered their heathen ways. When I met the man, he was in a retirement home, his body totally immobilized by arthritis except for his lips. I couldn't help thinking that if I'd had the power, I might have reversed the affliction and given him his mobility in exchange for arthritis of the lips. You see, he said to me, "I don't understand it. I served God for thirty-seven years, trying to make those people see the light, and now look how I'm rewarded." And I replied, "God didn't give you arthritis; you gave God arthritis." And I meant it.

We are representative of the universe, a part of the whole. If we allow ourselves, for whatever reason, to get arthritis and be immobilized, we affect everyone and everything beyond our physical bodies.

THE IMMUNE SYSTEM OF THE WORLD

Your health is important to the rest of the world. Are you your brother's keeper? Yes. But how? Not necessarily by making great sacrifices or doing acts of service. By maintaining your own health and youth, you can strengthen the immune system of the world. And that is a blessing for everyone on the planet and for the whole universe.

2

SELF-REGULATION
AND
SELF-HEALING

The exciting message I can share with you is that there is not a single person in this world who does not have the ability of self-regulation and self-healing. It is marvelous that I am not alone, but most of us have not become aware of our ability. We have chosen by ourselves to come to this earth, and we are indeed creating our own reality. Therefore, our health is our own doing. When the Scriptures talk about God and the universe and omnipotence, they are referring to us and our potential. Yet instead of believing in ourselves, we still look to others to do it for us. People observe me demonstrate putting a needle through my arm, and some faint or experience pain in their own arms. They say to me, "Well, you can do it. You were born that way." I reply, "It's true, I was born that way. But you see, so were you."

Every baby has an instinctive sense of what it needs to be healthy. Just try giving a baby cold milk to drink. The baby won't swallow it, but will play with it, blow bubbles with it, and mix it with its saliva. Babies know by instinct that the acid in the mouth is the first stage of digestion and that the milk must be warm for this process to work. As adults, who use logic and reason, we drink a glass of milk right out of the refrigerator. The cold milk hits our glands and paralyzes them, and we end up with a spastic colon.

But we can regain the inner knowing we had as children. The evidence of our latent power for self-regulation is all around us. There was a woman in Germany, Theresa Neumann, who did not eat or drink for sixty years. Careful investigation by doctors and priests verified that the only thing she ever ate was the holy host at communion. She was very religious, and on every anniversary of the crucifixion of Christ, her hands, feet, and forehead would bleed.

I have seen others do similar things under hypnosis. If I place my finger on the forehead of someone in a trance and suggest that my finger is a burning cigarette, a welt will appear on the skin. If I give a hypnotized man a glass of mineral water and suggest that it is vodka, not only will he act drunk, but his blood alcohol level will actually increase.

In several scientific studies of placebos, control groups have showed higher rates of healing and recuperation than the groups taking the real medication. At our Aletheia H.E.A.R.T. Center in Oregon, we do something similar with the technique of perceptualization. For example, we let people perceptualize aerobics. We put a picture of someone doing aerobics on a screen. The people gaze at the screen for a while, then close their eyes and imagine themselves on the screen, doing the exercises. Physiological instruments show that their bodies respond as if they actually were performing the exercises.

If you had been with me on the battlefield in World War II, you would have seen that many people were shot and never noticed it or felt pain. Their wounds healed while they were doing what they needed to do to survive. In 1940, a hospital in Rotterdam was bombed. The ceiling caved in, the windows shattered, and flames leaped up. Patients, some of whom had been lying in bed for ten to fifteen years, suddenly jumped up, pulled out their tubes and wires, and ran in their bare feet over broken glass and through the flames to get outside. Not even their nightgowns were scorched. Each of them had the capability for self-healing, just as all of us do today. Do we need to get bombs in our hair to start realizing our potential?

So you can look for heroes, compare yourself with them, and sit at their feet in adoration, believing that they were born with all their abilities intact. You can search for the fountain of youth or a new herb you can take faithfully every day. But if you don't see that it is *you* yourself, your mind, your beingness, your spirit and pure energy that has the power, then you won't understand.

Self-regulation and self-healing is attained by becoming aware of our own energy transformations every fraction of a fraction of a second, not just once in a lifetime. We must learn to be excited, to make all our senses acute to our inner being. We need to stimulate the flow of the universal energy within us, without conscious control.

People sometimes say, "Jack Schwarz has pain control," as though I can consciously think away pain. The truth is I do not "control" the pain. Instead I identify with my higher nature; I expand my energy and, thereby, my consciousness. I set free energies that were contracted by stagnation. That is what releases me from pain. This expansion and release has nothing to do with conscious control. It is voluntarily allowing the body to regulate itself without interference.

To understand self-regulation, we must learn to recognize the true nature of our essential beingness. For a long time, I used to ask myself, "Who am I?" I finally gave it up. I saw that the Los Angeles telephone directory listed thirty-five Jack Schwarzes. Thank God I knew my telephone number; otherwise I would not, to this day, know which of the thirty-five I was. *Jack Schwarz* was clearly just a name, and not a very unique one. I stopped asking, "Who am I" and started to ask, "*What* am I?" Then I realized I am not just this body that I look at in the mirror, not simply flesh, blood, organs, bones, hair, and skin. I am energy. In fact, as Martin Buber, the Jewish philosopher, points out in his book *I and Thou*, what I really am is a part of the universal energy that exists in all of us, and which will continue to exist long after the vehicle—my body—is in the wrecking pile. Energy is the transpersonal self that trusts the I-self, the Jack Schwarz–self, the body-self, to do the job. Knowing this, Jack Schwarz can stop telling the body what to do. The body is very wise. Its involuntary processes, with proper direction of the mind, can give you the capacity to regenerate cell for cell.

When I was at the Menninger Foundation demonstrating my ability to put needles in my arm without bleeding, some of the assistant researchers asked me, "Jack, how does that feel?" I answered, "Let me check with my body. Let me ask my body how it feels." I had to start paying attention to my body, because, in a way, I was not putting a needle in *my* arm, but in *an* arm. I was saying to myself, "I'm the driver, and this is being done to my car, my vehicle, my instrument of expression." I was nonattached to my body, totally beyond the physical structure.

The scientists studying me learned that my body was in a state of relaxed awareness. Many people think relaxation means to become a Raggedy Ann, but you can be relaxed and at the same time highly energetic. The answer is confidence: being absolutely nonattached, knowing that you are in that high-powered state and that you are in charge. Physiologically, this is a state of excitement throughout the body. The natural opiates in the brain, the endorphins and enkephalins and dopamine, are activated. At the same time, the pineal gland, which regulates the metabolic process, activates enough oxygen and glucose to maintain rational function and awareness.

It is our constant interfering with the body, based on belief systems, that stops self-regulation. By belief systems, I mean the assumptions, prejudices, and pronouncements of scientific authorities that too often pass for wisdom in our world. These belief systems mislead us from the moment of our conception. We come into our family belief system, and if we mature out of that, we get into society's belief systems and education's belief systems, which are all based on external knowledge. We start taking knowledge as the source for our growth, rather than as a tool, even though it is still based on other people's authority. As long as we rely on other people's authority, we will never find our own inner authority. We need to look each other in the eyes as equals. Your inner authority is as good as anyone else's.

How many times have you come home and someone says, "Oh, did you cut yourself?" Then they point to an injury you hadn't even noticed. Immediately, the cut starts hurting and you cannot wait until somebody brings an ointment. They tell you it might be infected and that you had better get a tetanus shot. You were doing fine until someone called your attention to it and got you to start following belief systems instead of your inner knowing.

I grew up in a home where my mother was bedridden, diagnosed with tuberculosis. She made sure that I had a checkup every three months, and I was told all kinds of things to do to avoid getting sick. In particular, I was warned not to get my feet wet.

We lived in Holland, and my house was in the middle of the meadows, which were surrounded by canals. We had roadways to go to school, but no self-respecting Dutch boy would go to school over the roadways. He would go through the meadows and jump the canals. I was told, "Now be careful, Jack. If you get wet feet, you will get tuberculosis." And I was given special socks that covered my legs all the way up to my hips.

The moment I was outside the house, I rolled these

girlish socks down so that I would not look foolish to the rest of the boys. Then I would jump the canals. Of course, for every hundred times I jumped, ten times I made it across and ninety times I landed in the canal. When I came home at night, I knew my family was going to feel my feet to see if they were wet and, if they were, I would be rushed to the doctor. So I had stolen a pair of socks and hidden them in the toolshed. As soon as I got home, I took my wet socks off and put my dry socks on. Then I came into the house and offered my feet for inspection. Since I had dry feet, my family was satisfied that I would not get tuberculosis.

You see, I was indoctrinated into belief systems like everyone else—do this, do that, don't do this, don't do that. I was constantly warned about all the bad things that can happen to us in daily life. We are encouraged to drive with one foot on the accelerator all the way to the floorboard, and the other foot on the brake to make sure that we hold back. Then we are surprised when the pistons don't work and the engine burns out.

But I discovered through my inner knowing that all these things I was being told were not true. My higher beingness told me that I would not be affected by anything that I did not allow to affect me. My inner knowing told me to stay in a constant state of high energy, to be excited by everything, so that I would keep my energy flowing. I could acknowledge and respond to things, but I didn't have to accept that anything would necessarily have an inappropriate effect on me.

I also discovered that we do not need to eat three meals a day to be healthy. There was a time when I ate only three meals a *week*, and each meal was only a handful. Eighteen hours working, two hours sleeping, and I was as healthy and as peppy as I could be. My body didn't ask for food because it was eating from the environment all the time. I have nothing against the middle men, the retailers, we might say, but sometimes I prefer to get my nutrition wholesale or from the source. It even gets delivered to me!

With my inner knowing, I learned that we can actually photosynthesize like plants. The more I live in a state of joy and excitement, the more all the particles in my body—the calcium, selenium, lithium, magnesium, phosphorus, and so on—get sparked and become ionized. These particles radiate energy and resonate with the ions in the universe, which I can then grab and use. That is my food.

So, believe in yourself and your own capacity for self-regulation and self-healing. You can't get it from others—not even me. I have been called a healer since I was nine years old, but, in truth, I haven't healed anyone except myself. And for all the self-healing I do, I am not invincible. The best I can do is exemplify the willingness to live to the fullest, to keep my generator going and my battery full. Other techniques such as herbs, medicine, homeopathy, and acupuncture may help too, but ultimately it is the person who heals himself. I am surely not a martyr or a savior or a guru. I only share what I have discovered in my own life. It is not the only way, but it may stimulate you to start changing your belief systems into knowing systems. Then you can start expressing that power within you.

We can help each other by maintaining our radiance, our health, so that energy is available for whomever comes into our presence. Sometimes people think they lack the energy to self-generate. They feel as though they are stalled in the middle of a road in the Sahara. Even so, they have a generator with which they can regenerate their battery.

Each of us can be like a cosmic AAA. We can drive over God's highways, and whenever somebody's car is stalled, we can stop and get out our jumper cables. We keep generating, keep our own foot on the accelerator and ask them, "Please put your foot on your own accelerator, too. Try it out now. Are you running? Fine. Goodbye!" And we go to the next one. You see, you cannot give your energy to anyone, but with your high energy you can surely activate their low energy.

You can help them to start regenerating themselves, and that's really called healing.

Learning self-regulation and self-healing is like creating a map of your inner being. You may find that there are a lot of people making maps, but you have to be careful. Unless they have walked the territory, the map has very little value. And even if they have, unless you experience the territory yourself and make your own map, you can still become quite diseased.

Sri Aurobindo, the Indian seer and poet, says, "You cannot relate to anything you don't know. You cannot know anything unless you can become it." No one can tell you how to heal yourself.

Sometimes people use a rigid discipline as their map, but discipline should not be punishing or restrictive of your inner spontaneity. Martin Buber, the author of *I and Thou*, tells a story about discipline. A young man was once sent to fast in the desert by his teacher. When his fast was nearly complete, he came to an oasis with a beautiful spring welling from the ground. He was so thirsty that he fell to the ground to drink, but just as the water was about to touch his lips, he decided, "No, I'm not going to drink. I'm not going to break my fast. I will discipline myself and do without water." But as he walked away, he realized that he was filled with a smug pride, which was as much of a stagnation as hate or anger. He then ran back to the spring and drank, knowing that it was better to break the fast than to stagnate the energy.

The root of the word discipline means "to be a disciple of." It follows, then, that we should be a disciple of no one but our higher self, our inner knowingness—a disciple of the Thou-self, which is resonating with truth from a higher level, rather than a disciple of only the I-self, which often gets sidetracked by the belief systems of our society.

To make a map for myself, I had to trace back in my body (a thinking, feeling, and knowing) the effects of the experiments I was performing on myself. When I was doing this research, people said to me, "You're doing something very unusual," or "Jack, that's very unnatural." I was often upset by these remarks because I felt that I was the only one who was really doing natural things. Everyone else was being unnatural by denying their own potential to do what I was doing.

Self-regulation and self-healing require that we take responsibility for our health. We can always find someone or something to blame, but we allow events and situations to happen to us. We are the only ones who can make changes. All the friends and lovers, all the belief systems in the world, may try to guide us and give us insights. Ultimately we have to do it ourselves. But responsibility does not mean feeling guilty for our mistakes. It means the ability to respond to our spontaneous insights, to our inner experiences. It means being able to articulate our insights and put them into practice, to dare to take action.

This cannot be done with just a single method. It has to be adapted to each individual's need and how a person's energy is flowing or not flowing. Therefore, we cannot copy someone and say that this is *the* method. There are gorgeous methods in some of my books. Fantastic techniques. As soon as you read them you may get excited and believe these techniques are the finest in the world. However, very quickly they can become detrimental to you because too many of us want to become technicians. When we start following techniques, we get so involved in the technique that we lose any sense of our own inner being. We begin to operate mechanically, not realizing that the technique should have been surpassed a long time ago.

Techniques are useful to show us where the jumper cables are to get things started. They are not meant to be hung on to, because hanging on to a technique can stagnate us. We should become less technique hungry. It is all right to find a technique, but we should then adapt it to our own beingness. Then we can have a good marriage between technique and inner being.

You don't have to die to become a saint. By that I mean that to the ones we call saints, the inner knowing and self-regulation by which they achieved ecstasy were parts of a normal life. They were living as we all can, they were not special chosen ones.

If you want self-regulation and self-healing, you must be willing to take risks and accept the consequences. The consequences are happiness and a healthy life. Is that so hard to take? Sometimes I wonder!

3

HUMAN
ENERGY
SYSTEMS

Human energy systems refer, of course, to the energy that we utilize while we are in a physical existence. This sounds like we are separating human energy from the energy of the universe, but it would not be appropriate to make such a distinction. Human energy systems are only forms of the universal energy as it exists in human beings.

In my classes and seminars I quite often tell people that, if I ask a question and they don't have the answer, they should just say, "energy" and they will always be correct. There is nothing in this whole universe that does not consist of energy in its many different forms. This is the view of modern scientists, and, of course, the wise men of the past knew this as well as the wise men of today. The law of the universe is the law of energy transformation. Nothing stays in one form. Energy keeps transforming in order to fulfill its function in this universe.

It is the same with us. We use the energy of which we consist to fulfill our functions. Each of us has a specific function. That is why we are also unique. Each of us has a specific level and pattern of energy, which can be similar but never exactly the same as that of another person. So it makes very little sense to compare yourself and your energy to anyone else's.

To understand how the universal energy operates through me, I imagine a circle, which represents the universe. This circle is without beginning, without end, and it is filled with energy. I like to think of the universe as a package of energy, a container that holds in that energy. The container is the universal soul, which contains the essence. It is us, all of us.

All of the particles in that energy container are following the law of transformation; they do not need to be goaded by anything. In our lives, in order to follow a law, we need to have a mental capacity, intelligence. We learn to follow the laws of our society and country, whether or not we study them in books. How? It is because we have intelligence. Intelligence, if we go deeper, is related to our conscience—our level of ethics, of morality. But following a law is based on how much intelligence we have.

The particles that exist in the universe—the electrons, neutrons, protons—keep moving without being told. We must assume that they have an intelligence, too—different from ours, because we are a compound intelligence of all the particles. Each particle that exists in us, or each "us" that compounds these particles, must have that level of intelligence. Otherwise, this morning when you got out of bed, you would have gone outside and screamed to the universe, "Please, electrons, protons, neutrons keep moving, because if you guys stop, it's the end of the universe!" But you knew they would, no matter what. Your body functions the same way; you don't need to tell it what to do. So we must realize there is a universal mind, a universal intelligence. The Tibetans chanted *Aum* out of their awareness of the all-universal mind. Later, this became "Om," the universal sound.

Somewhere in this universal container of energy, you exist. You are an individualized amount of energy in the universal soul. The moment that energy individualizes itself, it is an individual soul.

Imagine that the universe is like a bowl of water, where all the particles know exactly what to do. If I take a cylinder and put it right in the middle of the bowl of water, what happens? Is the water any different inside the cylinder than outside the cylinder? There is one difference: the water inside the cylinder is temporarily cut off from communication with the rest of the water. In the same way, some of the universal energy becomes individualized. Then you are temporarily cut off, unaware of what is happening outside the cylinder of your individualized mind. If you are in a room with other people, and I put a cylinder over you, you would be temporarily out of touch with the others. You would lose awareness that there are others in the room, too. First, you are an "is-ness," until the mind gets involved; then you become an "I-am-ness."

The particles that make up the universe are active in a process of transformation. As they transform, they reach a new frequency, a new power, and they become radiant. The energy that was individualized gets activated and radiates beyond the cylinder, beyond the individuality. It makes contact once again with the total consciousness, the total universal mind, by resonance. Similarly, through activity human energy systems become more aware of the universal mind and how to resonate with it. That is what we call "evolving." As we start to activate our energy at one level, we radiate out onto the next level.

We could also call this process "expanding," because we expand our awareness as well. Consciousness, as a level of mentality, is an inherent quality of energy. We cannot expand consciousness without expanding energy, and we cannot expand energy without expanding consciousness. Ripples hit the shores of a pond and then bounce back out to where the rock fell in the water. The same thing is happening with our human energy, although we cannot see it as clearly. I may seem to be interacting only with people here in the United States, but my energy ripples out, and somewhere in Tibet there are people in tune with that. They do not know what I am doing or what I am saying, but they are being affected by it.

The more your consciousness is expanded, the more you will resonate with the appropriate energy field and affect all around you. This is how we are actually our brother's keeper. The more radiant you become, the more expanded energy you have, the healthier you are. Evolution goes on, constantly changing, appropriately utilizing the dynamic energy process. The energy that radiates from you is going to affect your fellow man.

If you absorb energy without expansion, then you affect people, too; you actually become contagious to your fellow man, even though no one may realize it. Sometimes we can be actually more polluting to the environment through our mental and physiological states than the smokestacks of factories. Mental pollution can be as bad or as influential on people as environmental pollution. Therefore, we must maintain a higher extension of our energy and keep the energy in its highest, most powerful state. There would be no need for training, or courses, or seminars, if people just understood that they could be radiant all the time by keeping themselves in a state of excitement twenty-four hours a day.

You can sense these energy levels. You can feel whether or not someone is involved, whether or not the energy is in motion—e(nergy) in motion(al): emotional. Try this little test with a friend. Close your eyes and try to feel your friend's presence. Have your friend sit still, then get up and walk around. Even if you can't hear your friend walking, you may be able to feel the movement, because you are feeling the energy. Most of us are sensitive to whether people are bored or excited. Even if they do not say anything, we can feel their withdrawal when they hold back their energy, and their return when they restore it.

All healers—medical doctors and practitioners of acupuncture, acupressure, polarity therapy, Reiki, you name it—are experimenting with methods of using this energy in an appropriate way. It has been noted that the human body is like a wet battery and a generator. The fluid in your body is in a dielectric, pH-balanced state, very much like distilled water. This "battery" will not lose its energy, but will charge and generate energy by maintaining a chemical and electrical balance. There also needs to be a mental and physical balance, a harmony. When we talk about the Harmonic Convergence, we are referring not just to the earth and the universe, the sun and the stars, but to each individual's mind and body converging to a harmonious state.

In the human body, our legs are the ground wires that ground us to the earth. Our hands are the two jump wires, so that whenever we need healing we can use these hands. The palm of the right hand is masculine and has a positive charge; the energy moves clockwise and is contracting. The left palm is feminine and has a negative charge; so it is expanding and moves counterclockwise. To do any healing requires both hands, just as we use both jumper cables on a battery, to maintain the balance. This way we avoid creating a short circuit, or overcharging one polarity higher than the other.

There is a simple way you can discover this for yourself. Put your right hand out as flat as possible, then put your left hand crosswise over it, about three to four inches above it. Already you can feel something like an attraction. Now, keep your right hand still and move your left hand clockwise over your right hand. Observe what you sense and how this feels. Stop for a moment. Then move your left hand counterclockwise over your right hand. Now, just for one moment, place both hands with the fingertips together, then pull them apart slowly and see what you feel between the two hands.

When you move your left hand clockwise, you may feel a resistance, as if it is being pulled to your right hand, and there may be a feeling of denseness. When you move your left hand counterclockwise, it may feel lighter, cooler, looser, and freer, because your energy is expanding and you are setting it free. Clockwise, you are creating a ball of energy like a material substance. Counterclockwise, you start to expand your energy and become spacey and, therefore, cooler.

Suppose that you have a sore knee, and that it hurts on the patella. You would probably go to a healer to remove the pain and to heal your knee. But, why should you go to a healer if you could heal yourself? After all, you have your own jumper cables with you. So, take your right hand, and hold it near your knee, but without touching your knee (there is no need to touch in healing). Take your left hand and put it straight underneath where your right hand is, again without touching your knee. Any way that is comfortable for you is fine. See if you can feel coolness between your hands and a warmth on top of the disk of your patella. Below your knee it may feel cool, too. Your left hand may feel warm on the top and cool on the bottom. Now reverse the positions of your hands. Your right hand may feel cool on the top and warm on the bottom. Normally, in a self-healing session you would spend three minutes with the right hand above where the pain is to contract the energy, then three minutes with the left hand to reverse the process and expand the energy. Even if you don't register strong sensations of warmth and coolness, your knee should feel different to you when you are through. It is just a matter of learning to recognize what you are feeling. Then you can realize that you always have your own healing power. You have your own first-aid kit with you, in your hands.

You can use this healing power to help yourself when your chakras and human energy system centers are not in balance and you do not have the time to do all your chakra exercises. States of imbalance are common because, as chiropractors have noted, very few people have a normal curvature to the spine. Most people have problems such as scoliosis or lordosis. So, whenever you lack the energy you need to do something, or you need to restore your energy because you have given off too much and you start feeling tired, you can restore and balance all your chakras in about six minutes doing a very simple thing. You can do it almost anywhere except maybe in a public place such as a restaurant or department store because people might misunderstand you.

You can do this sitting down. First, put the heel of your right hand against your sacrum, and let your palm and fingers slightly bend around your coccyx and buttocks, the gluteals. Put the palm and heel of your left hand exactly on top of your posterior fontanel.

That is the crown of your head where the hair starts to spiral out, because it is affected by the ray entering there. Now, sit or walk, keeping your hands where you've placed them, for about three minutes. Then, reverse your hands. Put your left hand against the base of the spine, your right hand on your crown, and sit or walk for another three minutes.

Doing this exercise makes the energy move back and forth through your spine. When I do this, I can make my forehead become very cool or very warm. My standard joke about this is that when I go camping, I do not take my Coleman stove with me. If I want my eggs fried, I only have to put them between my hands on top of my head. I can get it so hot that I could fry my potatoes and eggs and toast my bread. The energy moving through my spine comes out of my forehead as heat I can feel, and my hand becomes hot. When I reverse the flow, my tailbone gets that hot, because I am pushing the energy down and my hand picks that up.

The energy moving back and forth through my spine has so much force that if I do this often enough, it can even straighten out my curvatures. Whenever I have a neckache or backache this method can immediately restore the balance within six minutes.

By the way, most pain in the neck is caused by your sensitivity to other people. People become a pain in your neck. When you lower your energy, when you are not radiating energy, then their energy becomes overpowering and affects you. It actually becomes your pain in the neck, with all the familiar symptoms. The first sign you get is a little churning feeling, a little nausea. The energy comes up and it starts to move above your brows, tightening them up. You can feel the pressure, and then it starts to radiate out over your skull and eventually into the occipital area, and then over your neck and shoulders.

When you get affected emotionally, but you cannot do anything about it, this energy starts to pile up, starts to churn. You do not let it out because you have learned to control yourself, control your anger. Of course, what you call "control" is really repressing your energy instead of controlling it. It tries to get out through the crown, but it is too material, too dense, like molasses, to get out there. Instead, it fills the cavity of the skull and it tries to get out through the fontanel. But at the back of the neck the psychic force is trying to get in, so there is a collision. The energy radiates out over the neck and the shoulders and that is where your pain in the neck comes from.

You can help yourself with neck pain by using your "first-aid kit." Put your right hand on your solar plexus instead of on the lower back. Put your left hand on the back of the head, with your little finger resting against the occiput, the atlas. Sit for three minutes that way and then three minutes with your hands reversed.

The pain in your neck will be released until you allow it to build up again.

I would like to go through another pain-control exercise, which you can do any time at home. Every time it will be a different experience for you. We call this exercise "drawing out your pain." I use the phrase *drawing out* both figuratively and literally.

I did this exercise once with the SAGE (Senior Actualization and Growth Exploration) geriatric group in Berkeley, people from 73 to 103 years old. I asked them, "Where is the pain?" Of course, among the 275 people I saw 550 hands go up—they all had more than one pain. I think if they had been a little bit easier on their feet, they might even have put their legs up too, to show there were more than two pains. Then we had them do this exercise, and we found that they got some good results, diminishing the pain and sometimes being released from the pain.

Take a sheet of paper and a box of crayons. Open the box, but do not look at it. Now, make yourself remember where the four corners of your page are. Those corners are the four places you will use. You are going to work partially with your eyes closed and partially with your eyes open.

Check within yourself if you have any pain. If you do not, then just imagine a pain or even reexperience a pain that you've had before. Evaluate the intensity of that pain—whether it is severe or just slightly pain-

ful, or somewhere in between. Do not necessarily identify the cause of the pain. In the first place, I would
like you to learn that in reality pain is not taking place
in your body, but is actually a disturbance, like a short-
circuit, in your energy field, which is then transferred
by absorption into the body. It is only your belief
systems that make you locate the pain in your body.
Also, realize it does not have to be a physical pain—
it can be an emotional or mental pain—something
that really bugs you and gives you the feeling of being
hurt.

Once you have established a specific pain, close
your eyes and take your box of crayons in your hand.
Without looking, pick out one crayon. On the upper-
left corner of your page, draw your pain, with your
eyes closed. Just spontaneously draw whatever comes;
make an effort not to think. Now put your crayon back
into your box. Open your eyes, but do not pay attention to what you drew or what color you used.

With your eyes open, take from your box of crayons a color that you feel best represents the state of
your being, as you are at this moment. If you had a
pain, and the pain is still there, then pick the color
that represents the intensity of the pain. If you do not
have a pain, then pick the color that represents you
as you are now. In the upper-right corner, draw your
feeling, or what you perceive. You can look at it if
you want, but you do not have to. Again, do not try

to make a picture. Spontaneously draw what you feel. You may want to number your drawings.

Now close your eyes again and pick a crayon without looking at it. Draw in the lower-left corner what you are experiencing. When you are through, put the crayon back, and open your eyes again.

With your eyes open, without thinking, try to pick the crayon that best represents your state at this moment. With your eyes still open, draw in the lower-right corner the state you feel you are in, what you are experiencing now. Again, you don't have to create a work of art, just a spontaneous expression. Put the crayon back. That is the end of the exercise.

I will show you how I interpret this exercise by going over some of the kinds of drawings people in my courses at the Center produced.

One person's first drawing, with his eyes closed, was a bluish-green line. To me, this had to do with an emotional state involving willpower. It did not represent a physical pain, per se, although it affected his body and he indeed hurt physically. The second drawing, with his eyes open, had more movement, which told me that his willpower had started to diminish and then expand—a growth process. His drawing also gave me a sense of which parts of his body were affected. The third drawing, with his eyes closed again, was a black starlike shape. Black told me he was absorbing energy; the star shape meant he was also alternately projecting energy but bringing it from a dense state into a wider state. His fourth drawing, with his eyes open again, was an elliptical spiral, which expressed expanded consciousness. I suggested to him, based on these drawings, that his pain was, if not totally gone, diminished by at least 95 percent. This was, in fact, what he had experienced. If I had not known him and he had just sent me these drawings, I would have been able to find out the same things.

For another person, the first drawing also indicated an emotional pain affecting the body, particularly in the solar plexus area. Her second drawing, with eyes open, indicated an effort of will to deal with pain that had been there for a long time. Her third drawing, with eyes closed, was an expanding ellipse, showing emotion in the heart that was becoming part of her consciousness. Her pain started to diminish as her consciousness expanded until eventually it was integrated with her activities so that it did not hamper her.

Another person's first drawing was orange—a pain of the heart in his consciousness. His second drawing, with eyes open, was greenish. This meant he became emotional about it, but it was also light; he had some intellect coming into play. His third drawing, with eyes closed, was a red figure spread across the whole width of the page. His pain became more vital, powerful, more fiery. At the same time, he really let go of it. He pushed a power behind it. In his fourth drawing, he had the blue of willpower, but it was now wavy like water. This indicated also that the energy was moving like water. At the end he became a little bit emotional, but it was willed away. The very real pain he had experienced at the beginning of the exercise was now practically gone.

In one session, a person's first drawing, with his eyes closed, was white, which indicated no pain, but that his mind was saying, "There might be pain here, but I am not going to pay attention to that. I am out there somewhere, and that pain will take care of itself." This was a slightly masochistic way of dealing with the pain. In his second drawing, with his eyes open, he started unconsciously to reason, "Well, I have the pain, but the pain is after all for growth. I will turn my energy into motion." In his third drawing, with his eyes closed, he expressed, "I am going to integrate this pain, make the pain useful in my life." He was using his mind to control the pain. His final drawing was a purple circle—without beginning, without end—which said, "My higher self is dealing with it." This was a man who a week earlier had hurt his knee so badly he couldn't walk. In the session, his mind did not want to recognize the pain or have anything to do with it. But through the exercise his unconscious said, "Okay, you bound yourself up again; if you don't want to walk, that's okay; we'll let you fly."

As you see, color is very important in this exercise.

Each color has a specific quality of power and relates to a musical note and key. When white is mixed with a color, the result is a pastel with greater power, and a musical note of a higher octave. In books about the human energy fields, you might sometimes read that a person who has pastel colors in his or her human energy field is debilitated. That is nonsense. White is all power; it is the whole spectrum. How can it be debilitating? It makes the color more powerful. I also see white as a reflection of light and, therefore, spirit or truth—universal truth.

Red is the musical note C. The more white mixed with red, the higher an octave C becomes. Red is the power, the energy field, the quality of vitality—life-promoting, life-activating. Pink is, of course, very high C. It also represents the life and love energy. People who go on a vegetarian diet often start out eating nothing but green salad three or four times a day. They do not study vegetarianism, and they do not include pigmented vegetables in their food. The more they eat greens, the weaker they become; they do not get enough light-promoting energy.

Orange, which is red and yellow together, is the color of intuitive consciousness. The more white in it, the higher the pitch, and the more gold it becomes. Gold represents the paraconscious mind and the musical note D.

Yellow stands for mental, intellectual energy and

the musical note E. Green is the most emotional, life-preserving power. It is in the key of F, and represents the regulation of emotion. Blue is in the key of G and represents willpower. The lighter the blue is, the more it is "Thy will be done." The darker the blue is, the more it is "My will be done."

Beethoven wrote nine symphonies and yet he was also almost deaf. He played by sensing rather than by hearing or seeing things. His sixth symphony, called the "Pastoral," is written in F major, which represents green, the emotional. When you listen to the "Pastoral" you hear nature: green meadows, forest, flowers. His nine symphonies are written in every key of the musical scale except one. He did not write any symphony in G. He did not have the blue, the power of volition.

The most musically pure tone is the note A, which is indigo. Indigo is actually three primary colors, equally blended together. It is hard for artists to make indigo, because they do not have the exact proportions of primary colors.

If we have three glass lenses of yellow, blue, and red on top of each other, we get opaque black—total absorption of light. The primary colors reflect the whole spectrum, but also have the capacity to absorb, in which case we see black. That is the synthesizing power that puts things together. It deals with the whole spectrum, not with the separate colors.

Finally, there is purple, from red and blue. The

vital, life-promoting power comes together with the willpower, and becomes integrated. Purple represents the musical note B.

Sometimes you pick the color of your clothing or your environment in order to nourish the needs of your body and mind. In nutritional evaluations I suggest food groupings based on color. I separate the green-blue vegetables from the pigmented ones—the whites, the reds, the yellows, the oranges, and the purples. I suggest that when a person is low in energy they should eat 65 percent pigmented vegetables and only 35 percent green ones. If a person is hyperactive, I suggest eating 65 percent green and only 35 percent pigmented vegetables. In this way you can also start to recognize that the colors have energy capacity and power.

Green-Blue Pigmented Vegetables
(one to two cups per serving)

Asparagus

Avocados (one-half)

Parsnips

Mushrooms

Cucumbers

Parsley

Broccoli

Green Beans

Brussels Sprouts

Cabbage

Kale

Lettuce (Loose Leaf or Bibb)

Green Peppers

Spinach

Red-Orange-Yellow-White
Pigmented Vegetables
(up to one cup per serving)

Cauliflower

Onions

Kohlrabi

Rutabagas

Beets and Beet Greens

Radishes

Red Potatoes

Potatoes

Garlic

Turnips

Tomatoes

Red Chile Peppers
(canned ok)

Red Cabbage

Yams

Sweet Potatoes

Eggplant

Carrots

Pumpkin and Yel-
low Squash

Red Peppers

Corn

4

THE
MOVING
MOMENT

We have been born into a time of world transition. Never in history has so much energy in so many forms been available. Never has information flowed so quickly. This is a privilege, but it may also feel oppressive or frightening. The accelerating pace of global change means there is less time to think through our decisions. The lessons of the past are less useful. Predictions of the future are less reliable. More than ever, we live in the excitement and challenge of a continuously renewing present—in the "moving moment."

It is astounding how rapidly things are changing. We have gone from wagon wheels to satellites in the sky in the span of sixty-some years. When I was born, we used candles and kerosene to light our houses. Then we went to gaslight. Then electricity came along. Now we are in the Information Age, and to communicate with someone around the globe may take only seconds. In this age of information, highly specialized knowledge quickly becomes obsolete. Human needs and desires fluctuate so rapidly that sometimes a product is outdated before it gets on the market.

Even our bodies are changing. When I was a young child in Holland, once a year my family went to the beach for two or three days. That trip of fifty-four miles was planned a year in advance. And at the beach if there was one man who was not covered with body hair, he was considered an oddity. Now, only sixty years later, if we see a man covered with hair, we call him a gorilla. Even in this short span of time, we see the human body evolving beyond a need for this protective coverage.

In a climate of rapid change, there are no final solutions, no sure ways to measure gains and losses or evaluate achievements. What you lose today, you may gain ten times over tomorrow. An act that seems terrible may have benefits that become apparent ten years from now. As Kahlil Gibran says in *The Prophet*, "Your joy of today is your suffering of yesterday unmasked."

There are no longer absolutes in knowledge or experience. I remember being taught in school that nothing can travel faster than the speed of light. Yet today scientists theorize tachyons, particles that travel faster than light. Cause-and-effect relationships must also be reconsidered. Just because a particular series of events led to a certain result in the past does not mean it will have the same result in the future. Even our personal value systems, once thought to apply to all generations, now call for constant reevaluation to remain relevant to our evolving conditions.

We can realize how blessed we are to be born in an age where everything is in a state of change. We are not mere witnesses, but active participants in the universe and its transformation of energy. However, adapting to constant change is not always easy. We do not give ourselves enough credit for how well we manage to cope, or fully realize how rough this has been for us. Many of us cannot move fast enough to keep up with the changing times. So we resist the pace of change, try to hang on to yesterday, and, as our energies stagnate, become prone to disease. Sometimes the pace seems relentless, forcing us to speed up continually. And it is only beginning. For the more we speed up, the more momentum our energies create, and the faster things will keep changing.

To find your place in a rapidly changing society, you need to remain flexible and roll with the changes.

It is much like being in an automobile accident: if you are relaxed, you are far less likely to be injured. But this means that we don't have as much time to hesitate or plan things out. We cannot constantly cram our heads with thoughts like Rodin's *The Thinker*. We must be alert for changes taking place and immediately adapt ourselves. We can't always wait a week, or a day, or even an hour, because by then the action we have planned may no longer be valid.

We must receive direction and information from an expanded variety of sources and avoid narrow points of view. This requires that we be aware of our inner lives, our intuitive knowing, so that we can resonate immediately with whatever comes at us. Resonance is the selective capacity to match ourselves—by activating all the particles in our bodies—to the exact frequency and amplitude of the radiant energy in our environment.

When we resonate at this level of consciousness, our senses awaken and we can see, hear, taste, touch, and smell with a higher sensibility. I call this total awareness of the energy within us and around us *perceptualization*. I deliberately use this word instead of *visualization*, which has become a popular tool in healing work. Most of what is being taught as visualization leads people to expect to visualize in the same manner that they see with their two eyes. But perceptualization is of a much higher order that shows us the essence of our being. It is to "see" fully with all five senses, even to the point of hyperaesthetics, meaning expanded sensory perception. This is the truth of the poets and philosophers of all ages, but many people still think higher vision is only a metaphor, not an actual sensory experience.

We can look at a couch, for example. Usually we see only its physical form. It is like glancing at the photograph of a couch in a catalog. We note its shape, color, and size. But we can learn to experience its essence. We can learn to see more than just the physical form of the couch as it is revealed by visible light. We can perceive all the electromagnetic fields that surround and permeate it. There is a way to experience the couch in which you can "see" the trees that became the wood used in its frame. You can "see" the steel that became its springs, the cloth that was woven into its fabric. You can be aware of the energy of every spot where the fabric is frayed or the springs are sagging from all the people who have ever sat on its cushions, or spilled something on it. Beyond all this, you can sense the undefinable, individual energy of the couch. You can perceive it as a unique, living being. Your senses can be aware of the energies of every particle in it. They have been brought together temporarily to be a "couch," yet each still on its own unique journey through the universe. You can even sense the oneness of the energy of all those particles with the energy of your own being.

This is to experience our perceptions holographically. A hologram is a pattern made by light in which each part of the pattern contains the information of the whole. In a similar way, each of our perceptions, even of something as simple and ordinary as a couch, can potentially allow us to experience the wholeness of the universe.

Our minds are continually perceiving, scanning the universe like a radar station. The pineal gland, between the two hemispheres of the brain, functions like a cathode ray tube that transmits and receives information to and from the universe. The highest amplitude and lowest frequency will be in touch with the most universal level of information. We draw this in, as an electronic pattern, just as a television set does. When we see a person on a TV screen, we realize we are not looking at the person, but at an electronic pattern on the screen that is in a state of continuous motion. Every movement the person seemingly makes on the screen is really the motion of the electrons. Although we cannot always perceive it, everything in life is also in this constant state of motion. Our minds and brains receive this information, and our level of perceptivity determines whether we have a clear image or a less clear one. Sometimes, like on a TV, our horizontal and vertical controls go out of adjustment, and we get confused!

The motion we see in the objects around us is of such a high frequency that they look as though they are not moving. Just as an airplane high above us in the sky may appear to be moving more slowly than a car on a nearby road, we are rarely able to perceive reality as it actually is. We have learned to conceptualize a three-dimensional world. Our brains immediately translate perceptions into conventional images with familiar associations. It is sometimes confusing to transcend our concept of a solid three-dimensional world and directly perceive the myriad energies around us. We think we are doing something wrong, rather than realizing we are perceiving at a higher level of consciousness.

Much of the time we let our concepts do our perceiving for us. We take in a small amount of sensory information, then our brains tell us what we're perceiving, and our bodies react to the images in our minds. I often tell the story of a woman who came to a counseling session. As soon as she entered the room, she noticed a bouquet of roses on my coffee table and immediately began to sneeze and cough.

"What's the matter?" I asked.

"I'm . . . I'm allergic to roses," she said.

"How fascinating," I responded. "You are allergic to silk roses as well!"

And then, the moment she realized the roses were not real, her allergy attack stopped. It's not always true that a rose is a rose is a rose!

This kind of narrow perception, based on past concepts and expectations, prevents us from directly experiencing what is really there in each moving moment. Only by perceptualizing—by living with our senses awakened in the present—can we respond intuitively and spontaneously to the demands of rapid social and personal change. That is why I stress perceptualization. With our senses asleep, we rely on our thinking and we become stuck in the past.

I would like to close this chapter with a few suggestions for how to stay in the moving moment. First, try to be less obsessively goal-oriented. In Western society we are taught from the time we are toddlers to set goals—usually ones already laid out for us. We are directed toward what our life should be with many "shoulds" and "should nots."

But rigid goals can be detrimental to our capacity to grow *toward*. Too often we think of a goal as something that locks us in to a specific concept or course of action. We often symbolize a goal with the graphic illustration of a box. Then we box ourselves in. We forget about change and spontaneity, and our projections, prayers, and desires become too structured and limited. For example, suppose you want love in your life. Instead of asking to give and receive love or to be allowed to love, you focus on wanting a slender lover with black hair and brown eyes. Chances are, if you put out a call to the universe for a slender, black-haired lover, that is what you will get. But you may not be open to love in another form and you may not find real love.

Aim is a more appropriate word than *goal*. When we aim for something, we are going after a moving target. Then we move with it. Conversely, it is difficult to aim at a stationary target when we know we must stand perfectly still, perhaps holding our breath, afraid that moving a single muscle will throw off our aim.

I endeavor to have everything in my life become a moving target. That includes personal relationships, business dealings, and my interactions with society as a whole. I try to become the perfect archer, gaining my strength from what I experience at the very moment. What is perfect? It is the best you can do at any particular moment, recognizing that in the next moment you will need to do better.

Second, to stay in the moving moment, try to go beyond specialization and become an all-around person. Look at all of your potentials. Overspecialization tends to make us narrow our perspectives and think that we can't do anything beyond our limited training. But you have the potential to do anything you want to do, to be anything you need to be. Ask yourself how often you have done something you've always wanted to do, even though it had nothing to do with your specialized training and you may have been told you "should not" do it. That openness and spontaneity is the key for flowing responsively with change. You can always find within yourself the ability to begin new behaviors. You never have to be stuck in a static image of yourself.

Finally, I cannot stress enough the importance of keeping excited. Try to live in what I call a state of progressive excitement. Let your energies be activated. Begin to use your emotions creatively. Even your anger can become a marvelous tool for releasing your kinetic power. Do something to impress yourself. Too often we do things to impress others, and we lose the joy of self-discovery. There is a great joy in realizing you do not need to suppress your energies. Don't let possessiveness or guilt over the past hold you back. This universe was not created "for getting," but "for-giving." Forgiveness means not holding on to anything, but letting it go the moment it has performed its function, giving it back to the universe.

Realize that there is not one single thing in this life that you cannot be excited about. Even when something goes wrong, it is a challenge to see if you can do something about it. When you feel tired, it only means that you have compacted your energy and are not permitting it to flow. Think of the many times you came home from work tired, but then something exciting happened. Suddenly you were not tired. Many times we are bored, and fatigue is an excuse to stop moving until something exciting comes along. If you are feeling low, you can always recall your most recent peak experience and use that feeling of excitement to generate energy. Or you can focus on something in the near future. For example, when I'm dealing with grief or somberness, I think about going to Holland to be with my relatives, who always welcome me, even pamper me. Don't limit yourself to only certain things you think are appropriate to get excited about. That kind of thinking stagnates your energy.

Excitement comes from accepting change as a challenge to your own personal growth. Some people find rapid change overwhelming. Others accept change as a fact of life, but complain about it as a burden. Don't wait for a crisis to arise as an obvious challenge. Instead, look on each moment of your life as a challenge. Can you find the excitement? What can you do right now that can make the next moment better? That is the challenge. In the Scriptures it is written, "The best is yet to be." I believe that is true, and that the crown of God hangs in front of our faces.

Sometimes we make a mistake when we label children "hyperkinetic" or "hyperactive" instead of accepting and guiding their excitement into more creative forms. Remember that children live wholly in the moving moment. You only have to look into the eyes of newborn babies to see not only joy and excitement, but a tremendous knowingness. Be sure that they are going to teach us something that all of us still need to learn.

5

FEAR
NOT

Fear is a factor that can debilitate us and retard the process
of change. It can literally inhibit the life force. Fear is in-
evitable for all of us. We can never deny the necessity for
fear any more than we can deny the necessity for pain. But
if we can learn to view fear as a challenge, a creative challenge
for change, we can transform a seemingly negative quality
into a positive one. Both fear and pain are actually warning
signals for us to become alert: changes are about to happen.
Fear is caused by our unknowingness, our lack of consciousness about what is trying to come forth. Fear is also an in-

dication that there is a disconnection, a separation between our conscious state of mind and what I call our paraconscious. Viewed from that perspective, fear is a necessary incentive.

When I look back on my life, I see many periods in which I had reason to fear the unknown. Four times, through acts of war, acts of man, and acts of God, I lost everything I owned except the clothes on my body. And they were not such great clothes either! I admit that at the time I didn't always have a high enough level of consciousness to say, "Wow, isn't that fantastic? I get a chance to start all over again." But now I feel very blessed that the universe helped me by not allowing me to become too attached to anything. It's clear to me that I had been indoctrinated by my environment to be too attached, and that I needed a push to change.

Changes can be stressful, and you have probably heard many people say that we shouldn't have stress. You may actually be afraid of stress, of being overwhelmed by pressures.

But stress is a necessity, a part of the law of life. Stress keeps you moving, keeps your energy going. If you try to shoot an arrow from a slack bow, it won't go very far. Facing stress and dealing with it can actually be a stimulant for you, if you do it with your own inner knowingness.

We need stress as a challenge. Remember those

75 trillion cells in our bodies? Between each cell there is an infinitesimal space and within that space is motion, a state of stress that keeps communication between the cells going. Imagine a group of people who have been picked by a computer for their compatibility. Do you think that much growth will come from that group? Rarely, because they are so similar. They have only the same things to exchange. There is no stress, no spark. Have you ever seen fire without first a spark?

Why, then, are we afraid of stress? One reason is that we often don't adapt ourselves to conditions, but try to avoid stress. Then we get no fire, miss the light, and have no energy to deal with stressful situations.

I have never learned from anything in life that went smoothly, and, in my opinion, too many people think that when things go smoothly, everything will be okay. I have learned more from adversity—not by trying to figure out what hard times will do to me, but by acting upon them. I have responded, not simply reacted, and I have always come out for the better.

Many people cope with their fear of change and the unknown by imagining the bad things that may happen to themselves and to the world. People expect me to sympathize with them when they are disappointed or dissatisfied and are disappointed when I don't.

The Sufis have a marvelous aphorism in which God

speaks to the things he has created. For instance, God asks the tulips why they are standing up so straight and by themselves. They say, "We're standing up straight because we like to make an empty cup of ourselves." Then he asks the coal why it is so black, and the coal answers, "Because I have absorbed all the sins of the world." Then God says, "What will be your punishment?" The coal replies, "I will be devoured by fire." "What will become of you then?" says God. "Well," says the coal, "under even more pressure I will become a beautiful diamond."

You see, we need to learn to be dependent upon our inner selves, and pressure helps. But we have to get into action, not reaction.

I know that there are teachers who create guilt by pointing the finger and telling people they should be responsible for themselves. Just remember that when you point a finger at somebody, three fingers are pointing at you; so you'd better keep your hand behind your back. I tell people to recognize their responsibility, but I don't feel guilty that they haven't done it sooner. If you are dissatisfied with yourself, remember that you are awake now and have started to act. You don't need guilt.

I can have self-expectations without guilt by considering myself a "dissatisfied content" person: by being simultaneously happy and unhappy with myself at this moment. I enjoy sharing with you now, but am dissatisfied because I know it is not my best yet. On the other hand, I'm very content because I know in my inner being that I'm doing the best I can for now. That may not be good enough two seconds from now, and my dissatisfaction will then be the incentive to do better. Remember what we mean by responsibility: the ability to respond spontaneously by acting, not doubting and fearing.

Instead of guilt, try humor. To be able to laugh at yourself is a necessity. If you laugh at yourself before someone else laughs at you, you actually take the wind out of their sails.

Sometimes I joke about buying a Nabisco factory. Then I can make just one kind of cookie to help all of you who want spirituality, a special kind of chip cookie. It won't be microchips, but spiritual chips, and only one brand: "Risk-it Biscuits." Then, whenever you feel doubt or inertia coming up, take a Risk-it Biscuit and off you go. I say that all diseases—and I don't care what label you give them—find their source in the fear of change, the fear to let go because we don't know what the next step will bring. I have never understood why we are so security conscious in this society. If you already know the results of what you are working for, where is the challenge? Where is the discovery? Where is the excitement? What if I were to tell you exactly what you were going to find under your Christmas tree? How much excitement would you have opening your packages? The fact that we don't know what is coming keeps us alert and energetic. The outcome of anything is never known in advance. The success you search for might be your own downfall if you attach yourself to the success. It can stagnate you and create inertia.

Sometimes people want to know what's coming because they are afraid of failure. This is another fear that stagnates your energy. But letting go of that fear allows you to stay activated and excited. When I started my Center, people began telling me that I was looking younger. I always responded, "Wouldn't you look younger if you fell on your snoot and got a nose job ten times a day?" You see, if you fail, it's a challenge. You get up and remember that you know how to walk and that you have to work to bring in excitement to keep things going.

We need to wake up. We cannot pick and choose any longer, hesitating out of fear of change or fear of failure. We must dare and risk, because our foundations are shaking and may crumble fast. We must change old belief systems into knowing systems. Fear can be used to our advantage. It tells us, "Aha! I need to deal with what is happening."

This does not apply just to certain individuals. All our lives are being changed, perhaps against our will. Nevertheless, change will make us more alert, more self-dependent. We will have to search the tool kits of our life to discover the tools we have available. This can be an exciting search, because most of us haven't even touched most of our tools yet. Most of our potentials have been denied. We are afraid of knowing ourselves, afraid of relying on our own inner authority. It is hard to look within ourselves because we can always get the answers somewhere else. We can pick a book or go to a lecture. We can take a class or talk to those who are seemingly successful. Instead of believing in our own experience, we still turn to others to ask, "Do you think I will be able to do that?"

How could anyone else know? The only one who can know is you—and you will know by doing. But you will never "do" if you worry about success or failure, or think you must know ahead of time what you're going to get. Let go of these fears: we get what we need. The Sufis have a marvelous saying: "My intuition never fails me, but I fail when I fail to listen to it." Too often we fail to listen to ourselves out of fear.

You know, you can always be certain of my loving you. But don't be terribly certain that I will like you, too—or like your behavior, or your resistance to change, or your dependency on those who have made changes, or the way you stop after a change and say, "Look, I just changed. That's how I did it"—without realizing you must continue to change.

A beautiful statement that has helped me a lot is "As long as you can find a place for one foe in your heart, it is a very unsafe abode for a friend." Now ask yourself what you call a foe. Personally, I call one little resentment a foe, or one little doubt, because resentment and doubt are foes of our creative capacity. They are enemies of our progressive, dynamic evolutionary state. It would not be safe for you to seek room and support in my heart if I still have one of these little foes living there. One foe can turn the whole environment around and make it an unsafe abode for anyone.

When you feel resentment or doubt, when you are afraid that you will never be loved by others, or you are afraid to accept that you are loved, it is only because you are afraid to recognize your love for self. I'm not talking about the body, this vehicle I'm driving. The body can do its job by itself, but only if I have enough self-love to allow it to take care of itself. Self-love is not egotistical, narcissistic love, but a radiant love of self, so radiant and exciting that you practically startle everybody, even in the most dreary circumstances. It is not simply that you walk with a smile on your face, but that your whole body smiles. Your being smiles like a spark of light in a dark hole.

We start going off the track when we are afraid we won't be accepted, when we need to belong, when we start to look for heroes. Did you ever consider that as soon as you are accepted by your fellow man, you are likely to be ignored? If you go through all kinds of game playing just to be accepted and loved, it won't work. However, if you radiate from your beingness, you will be acknowledged for whatever purpose you are here.

Did you know that an estimated 60 percent of medical patients are fearful that their cures may be successful?

We can help others only from a place of self-sufficiency. I am the authority only for myself. I can share my beliefs with you, but, for heaven's sake, don't accept a word I say until you test it within yourself. As a very young boy I discovered that we had many powers that I was told were impossible to have. I had to learn things for myself. You should do the same. When you feel that little "Aha, I know that" go off inside, that is verification that a statement or thought has value for you. For the rest, just throw it all in the first garbage pail you see and make sure that it gets recycled, because our universe is a biodegradable environment.

Fear of being ourselves keeps us from recognizing our own inner rhythms and harmony. To bring harmony to the world we must understand our individual inner beings and communicate—not simply verbally, but by daring to be what we are. You don't need to be afraid of what anybody thinks about you. You don't need to defend yourself, make excuses, or explain why you are the way you are. It's no one's business. You are what you are, and you can be so self-confident that you are completely harmonious within your own self.

If you want to become healthier, prevent disease, and bring about peace on earth, you have to allow yourself to be vulnerable. But vulnerability is another idea we fear. Society tells you not to be vulnerable, because if you are, all kinds of bad things will happen to you. Yet it is only by being vulnerable that the really good things can happen to you. Be spontaneous, be yourself, be vulnerable—even if you get kicked in the pants. We have been told this repeatedly over the ages, but we act as though we have never heard it.

Every true philosopher has said to turn the other cheek, but we don't understand. It does not mean that you should allow yourself to get hit or abused. It means that as long as you are afraid of being vulnerable, you will take offense at what people think or say about you and feel you must defend yourself. As soon as you are secure in what you are, you cannot be offended. Then you can allow yourself to be vulnerable. You know, from inside, that your energy field is so high that there is no way that a lower energy field can ever enter into it. You are not offended, and you have no need for defense.

Almost without exception we have an inner knowledge of these things, and yet it seems that something holds us back. We are conditioned to hold on, to be afraid to let go of what we know. We are afraid to risk losing what we have when we don't know what is ahead. Without vulnerability, we cannot be open to change.

I know all of us are afraid of pain, but few of us realize how much pain is caused by fear. You can think of fear as an alarm clock, and pain as the sound of the snooze alarm. If you don't wake up the first time you notice the fear, you'll get a little pain. You've had five minutes to wake up and you didn't. So now what do you do?

Often, instead of listening and saying, "Thank you, I'll get up now and take some action," we let the snooze alarm keep going. There must be something wrong with the clock. Do you hear that snooze alarm? This time it's called a headache.

Then we hang on and attach ourselves to the pain, not acknowledging that its cause is our underlying fear—our unknowingness, our not daring to risk or be spontaneous, not daring to be excited about something we've discovered.

Every day we have many opportunities for discovery. As we walk in our garden of life, there are all kinds of little green sprouts coming out. But we see one thistle and get totally stuck. We start asking all the neighbors, "Who put the thistle there?" And maybe we refuse to nourish all the other plants that are growing until we know who put the thistle there. If we can't find out, we call the whole block to go on a search party to find out why the thistle is there. In other words, we spread our grief and pain.

The thistle frightens us. Today it is one thistle; tomorrow it may be a dozen. Instead, the thistle is saying, "Get up! Do something! Don't allow the fear to become stuck in you."

When you respond to your pain and fear instead of ignoring them, you can start to unlearn the behaviors based on how you were told life was supposed to be, and you can begin to discover your own way. Life can become a series of continual, joyous discoveries.

For myself, I believe—and know deep inside me— that I deserve everything that happens to me. I think back to the time during World War II when I was placed in a prison camp. Initially, I had the reaction, how dare they! How could they put a good person in an environment like that and practically kill him. It was unheard of! That was where you put criminals and bad people—not good people like me! And yet, I now recognize that if it hadn't been for those terrible, negative five years of my life, I wouldn't be here sharing with you. In fact I wouldn't give a damn about you, because I was a narcissist. I was only after my own growth, bigger and better. I had to be stopped even though I didn't like it.

Many of us fear pain as an indication that we are not healing, but pain often means that we are interfering with our own healing process. Look at it this way. If you put all your financial resources into the stock market, you cannot have the same amount of money in your savings account. By the same token, if you put all your energy resources into pain, you will stagnate and inhibit your healing.

Pain is simply a part of the healing process that tells you something is changing within you. Pain is not even necessarily telling you that something is wrong. We need to be alert to pain without letting it stagnate us. It has the same purpose as those little lights on the dashboard of your car that tell you when your battery is weak, your water is low, or your fuel tank is empty. When you see one of those lights go on, you don't need to react by slamming on the brakes. You just know that it is saying, "Pay attention, fellow. Changes have to be made."

A person who has broken his elbow may have a cast for eight weeks, and when the cast is removed, he finds himself in a different situation. He must train his arm muscles to start moving again. The training may be very painful, but is he going to stop because he cannot stand the pain? No. If he lets the pain stagnate him, he inhibits his growth. And, of course, if he continues to train his muscles, he will move through the pain. Pain can be a friend if you don't permit yourself to be overpowered or impressed by it. Recognize it as part of a process and not as a detriment.

Death is part of the healing process, too, though we are usually too afraid to be conscious of it. At this moment, whether you like it not, we are all dying—including me. And thank God for that!

Who wants to live continuously with the same old cells year after year? By letting the cells die, you allow new cells to be born. This change needs to go on, because you can't function today as you functioned yesterday. Health is not a constant state, but a dynamic evolutionary process in which one second is never the same as the other.

You see, we have to make things "syntropic"—we have to start reshuffling the pieces and putting them together again without thinking, questioning, and doubting. Instead, we must dare to *be*, knowing that our inner being will tell us how. There is no book or tape or software available to tell us how it can be done. Don't expect me to tell you how! I can give you a clue, however. Start adapting yourself to the situation in which you find yourself without attaching yourself to it.

This may sound corny, but as afraid of death as we are, most of us have never said thank you for our life. We take everything for granted and allow others to tell us how to live. We strive for survival, but actually we value only physical survival. Yet mental, spiritual survival, which seems intangible, will continue to exist long after the physical. Your car will fall apart eventually whether or not you are attached to it. But imagine if you could say, "Thank God. Now I can get a different model!"

Each of us continues to go on after death, though not with our personality. The car is gone, but not the mind that helped it to drive over the road where it needed to go, the roads of life on this planet. That's why our personality is made up of the same stuff as this planet. That's why we have a relationship with the earth and are responsible for caring for it instead of robbing it and raping it.

This may sound harsh, but a lot of us are so fearful of life and so fearful of death that even though we wouldn't dare to commit suicide, we are doing it in a hidden way. I call it cellular suicide by not acting and thereby creating inertia, condensing and concentrating the cells and eventually creating ulcers or calcification or whatever physiological symptom you can find in the medical books.

We do not need to let fear make us unhealthy or kill us. We can go beyond fear and let out the potential that is within all of us for health, peace, and love. Those who have discovered their potentials and are using them are the ones who go ahead like scouts to bring back their discoveries to humankind—not so that others can follow, but so others can discover their own potentials within themselves. Then, we can go forward with one aim only: to know ourselves and be ourselves. Is that anything to be afraid of?

6

VOLUNTARY
CONTROLS

Voluntary controls is an approach to self-regulation and self-healing that works with levels of consciousness. We have different levels of consciousness that depends on the state of the brain, as identified by the types of brain waves—beta, alpha, theta, and delta. Brain waves are not actual waves of the brain itself, but an energy output of the brain that we can measure. If we could measure the energy inside the brain, it might be different from the brain waves.

It is helpful to think of the mind as being threefold, even though it operates as a totality. The outermost level is the conscious mind, the next level is the subconscious mind, and the innermost level is the paraconscious mind. Some people call this final level the superconscious, but I prefer paraconscious. The prefix *para* means beyond—beyond our personal consciousness.

The paraconscious is the level of the transpersonal, the universal, the divine. It is the level of the soul, the level of Martin Buber's "Thou"—the universal part of us that operates through a vehicle, the body, and through the outer levels of human consciousness, the conscious mind and the subconscious mind. The conscious mind is the level of the "I," your personal, individual identity and your outside perceptions as a physical self on this earth. The subconscious mind is an intermediate level of consciousness that functions as the archives and libraries of the mind. Everything that we experience consciously or unconsciously is registered in the subconscious mind and the energy of those experiences is always there, like electro-potentials in a computer. When we have the right frequency and the right amplitude, we can reactivate that energy, increase or decrease it. Sometimes we may get stuck, hammering away at the same material, trying to remember rather than reexperience what is in our subconscious mind.

We perceive through the conscious mind with the five physical senses, but every perception goes from the conscious mind to the subconscious mind, where it is compared with former experiences. After even a few years of childhood, what our senses perceive is based largely on preconceptions created from the experiences already registered in the subconscious mind. We verbalize these preconceptions as concepts, and if we have lived very much on the outside and have not dealt with our inner knowing, our inner world, and our intuitive beingness, we rely on those concepts instead of being open to new experience. To transcend the past, we need to activate the paraconscious mind, which perceives on a universal level of electro-potentials. The paraconscious is always a much higher power. It exists at the level of universal energy, more powerful than any limited earthly experience. It immediately transcends all that we have registered from the past.

Besides registering, administrating, and regulating experience, the subconscious mind is also charged with regulating the physiological actions of the body. This task takes a lot of energy. But if we tie up the energy available to the subconscious mind in the filing cabinets, archives, and library, we won't have very much energy for regulating the body. To have the power to drive it through, we therefore need to increase our amplitude, the voltage, in order to become powerful in our expressions and our experiences. One of the ways to do this is through breathing.

Since ancient times, breathing has been recognized

as one of the most important physiological actions on planet earth. As living beings, we need oxygen to be actively involved, to be alive. When we speak of the breath of life, we are not kidding. When someone's heart stops pumping, we know that within seven minutes the brain will die, so we have invented ways of blocking in the oxygen in the brain so that the brain cells do not die from lack of oxygen before the heartbeat has been restored.

The subconscious mind regulates our breathing so that we get enough oxygen in order to reach the different levels of mind together with different levels of body control. For this reason, we should give a lot of time and importance to breathing techniques.

Let me give you a metaphor for the attention we should pay to our breathing. I am driving a car and it suddenly stalls. Whatever I try, I cannot get the car to go. I might put the car in neutral, then get out, go behind it, and push. As soon as the car is rolling, I quickly jump back in, put the car into gear, and now I can drive. So I am actually pushing the car back into its function. While normally the car drives me, now I drive the car.

The same is true of breathing and the subconscious mind. My subconscious mind is like the car that drives my respiratory rate and thereby regulates my body. But if the subconscious mind is not functioning prop-

erly, then I might have to use my breathing to jumps-
tart it. Then I can put it back into the proper gear—
in this case, the proper brain wave state. You can think
of the different brain wave states, the frequencies and
the amplitudes, as the transmission of your vehicle—
your body—very much like the transmission gears in
your other vehicle, your car. The breathing exercises
help to jump-start the mind to operate again in specific
brain wave states, thereby regulating the body.

We must realize that there are many patterns of
breathing. Each pattern is characterized by how fully
we fill our lungs from the top down when we breathe
in air, and is associated with a brain wave state. If I
jumped at you suddenly, you might change your
breathing. Shallow breathing does not allow you to
get enough oxygen to the brain or to fill the lungs
sufficiently to get any power from them. So when you
are in a state of shock or panic, your breathing is
shallow and fast, and you feel paralyzed. We call this
clavicular breathing, or beta breathing. It fills the lungs
in the top only, without any intermission or holding
in, and the brain wave pattern is a very high frequency,
low amplitude beta state. There is no power, no voltage, to activate the body. If we are too expanded and
we want to ground ourselves, we might use this type
of breathing. We might do a couple of short breaths,
without holding in or holding out, in order to get the

feeling of the body back again, to purposely become more contracted. But, as a general rule, we do not want to breathe this way.

The next type of breathing is called intercostal breathing, or rib breathing. We put our chests out, and breathe through our chests. This does not fill the lungs very much—again, there is not enough power behind it. They teach you this particular breathing in the military, where you need your kinetic power, but you do not need any authority or mental power. This is still a type of beta breathing.

Next is diaphragmatic, or abdominal, breathing, which brings us into a slower rhythm with more power. This is moving the belly out to inhale, and back to exhale, using the diaphragm. It fills the lungs almost three-quarters full and is associated with alpha brain waves.

There is a slower abdominal breathing that we call theta breathing. It fills the lungs about seven-eighths full and is associated with theta brain waves. And finally, there is what we call paradoxical breathing, in which the belly goes in when we inhale. A newborn baby pulls in its belly for inhalation, and on exhalation the belly goes outward. When you put the baby on mother's chest, the baby starts to breathe like mother does, which is abdominal breathing—belly out when she inhales and belly back in when she exhales. Paradoxical breathing is a very slow, very long-lasting rhythm. It fills the lungs totally and is associated with delta brain waves. You should breathe this way only when you need to go into the delta brain wave state.

By changing the rhythm of our breathing we change our brain wave states and, therefore, our states of consciousness. Beta brain waves are associated predominantly with the conscious mind, alpha brain waves with the subconscious mind, and theta brain waves with the paraconscious mind. Since the subconscious mind regulates the body, the voluntary controls you exercise for healing and pain control take place in the alpha brain wave state. Every time I damaged and healed my body in the laboratory, all the instruments monitoring me showed that I was predominantly in the alpha brain wave state. Any time you need to do something with your body, you can use alpha breathing to jump-start the brain into the alpha brain wave state and activate the subconscious mind.

In beta breathing, you inhale, hold in, exhale, hold out. To go from beta to alpha, you inhale for a count of eight, hold for eight, exhale for eight, and hold for four. To go from alpha to theta, you inhale the same amount of air as in alpha but with a count of four, then hold for eight, exhale for eight, and hold for four. The pattern for full breathing is inhale for four, hold for eight, exhale for sixteen, and hold for four. To go from theta to delta, you inhale for four, hold in for eight, exhale for thirty-two, hold out for four. Any count over thirty-two on exhalation takes you to delta breathing. Some people can reach a pretty long exhalation. When I pay attention, I can reach a count of about 128 or 130 on exhalation when I want to go into delta. This may sound like a lot, but you can adapt yourself to it quickly. I suggest you put breathing exercises on a tape recorder with a timed space between exercises, so that each exercise takes half an hour. You do not need to count, since the tape counts for you. As with any type of exercise, the technique will interfere with the experience in the beginning, but after you train your unconscious mind, you will be able to use your breathing so that whenever you must respond to a situation, your unconscious will go automatically to the appropriate brain wave state.

Let us do several breathing exercises. The first one is learning to extend your exhalations in abdominal breathing so that you can go from alpha to theta. If you feel that you need to make sure that you are really breathing from your abdomen, you might want to put your hands on your belly and up on your kidney areas. To begin, inhale for a count of eight, hold in for eight, exhale for eight, and hold out for four. Do this three times.

Now inhale for a count of four, hold in for eight, exhale for eight, and hold out for four. Do this three times. Then try extending the exhalation. Inhale for a count of four, hold in for eight, exhale for sixteen, and hold out for four. Do this only once. Now, inhale for four, hold in for eight, exhale for thirty-two, and hold out for four. To do this, you must let the air go out so that the outflow is distributed over a longer time period. If you do not have any air left after a count of seventeen or whatever number you reach, then just start breathing regularly again; do not force yourself to reach the full count. If you reached thirty-two, try the exercise again from the beginning and see if you can reach an exhalation of forty-eight. You may find that each time you do the exercise, you can reach a longer count. With a little training you can reach forty-eight and further. Try this over several days. You will probably be able to extend your exhalations pretty quickly. In the beginning you might try to count too much, but it is just a matter of trusting that you will make it.

Here's another exercise that combines breathing and perceptualization. This is more than visualization; it is experiencing all five of your physical senses: smell, taste, touch, hearing, and sight. When I ask you to perceptualize, let yourself operate through whatever sense comes and see if you can also activate the other senses. But do not hang yourself up on one specific idea, trying to see or hear or taste it, and thereby using all your energy on that. Let what comes, come. Just be a very good observer of how it happens.

To begin, close your eyes and imagine that you have a blue cloud hanging in front of your head. Now inhale that blue cloud and, even though we know that your air goes to the bottom of your lungs, imagine that the cloud goes all the way down to the base of your spine. Exhale very slowly, and put the blue cloud outside of your head again. See what changes have taken place; perceive any differences in the cloud. Again, inhale the cloud, and hold it in; sense the cloud's being there at the base of your spine. Perceive if any changes have taken place. Check what changes and feelings you have inside your body. Observe, using as many sense perceptions as possible, what the cloud has become. Do it a third time. Inhale whatever is left of the cloud, hold it down at the base of the spine, and see what you can sense of it. Finally, let it go again. Do not pay attention to it any more. Just let it flow out. For the last time, observe what it has become. Do not pay attention to your breathing anymore; open your eyes.

Now, think about what you experienced. Perhaps you may imagine the cloud, make it blue, and it changes immediately into another color, or it never becomes blue, or it is never quite a cloud. If this happens, there is no reason to make an effort to see precisely a blue cloud. I have found that when I teach people an exercise, I am sensed as an authority, and if I say to imagine something blue, people make an effort to perceive blue because they think I must have a purpose for picking that color. But I just pick any color and wait to see what your own unconscious does. Your conscious mind takes my blue color, but then your unconscious decides it should be something else. Acknowledge that. It makes no difference if I had said make it multicolored. You have a good opportunity to learn about your own unconscious mind. I want you to realize that your unconscious decides what needs to be. You can consciously set up pink, and have it immediately become green. Allow it to become green then. The reason you might not be able to perceive the blue I suggested, even if you want to, is that your unconscious is stronger than my authority. Your conscious mind might be in charge of your perception for a fraction of a second and then it immediately changes to what your unconscious needs anyway. This type of exercise helps us become aware that the unconscious mind is stronger than the conscious mind.

During this exercise, you may have real physiological feelings. You may have a sense of losing your body. Do not be afraid it won't come back. This feeling happens because your consciousness is starting to become more affected by higher states of being. You always have your sense perception to restore yourself. If you come back very quickly, you might feel a little floaty or dizzy.

We can use these physiological changes to diagnose the needs of the body. For example, you might feel a slight movement in one area of your body, such as your back or hips, as if something were set free there.

Here is one last breathing exercise. Close your eyes again and perceptualize. Perceive your body with every pore as an entrance and an exit. Imagine when you inhale that you are drawing in through your pores. Feel all the air and oxygen going through the pores into your body. Now as you hold in your breath, command the pores to close. When you exhale, imagine the pores are open again. Exhale through all the pores.

As you breathe, keep your eyes closed and imagine all the pores, feel them, sense them with whatever sense perception you can use. Let all the air flow through the pores, very powerfully, then out of the pores. All the gates are open. Keep them open for a moment. Now again draw in all the energy, all the air, through every pore. The gates are open. Take it all in. Then close the gates, close the pores. Open them and powerfully exhale all the air through the pores and keep them open. Now inhale for the last time, powerfully. All the pores are now open wider. Let the air come all the way in. Now, for the last time, open all the gates and exhale all the air. Let your breathing restore itself without paying attention to it, and open your eyes.

You may have physical sensations during this exercise, such as heat, or you may feel pleasantly cool. You may perceive or feel you are in the light. I never suggest this beforehand, but there is always someone who feels a tingling like an electrical current, or like rolling through the snow. I feel it like the tingling after I give my skin a good brushing. You might just feel spacey, that is a sense of expansion, like floating. It is like less pressure, like a lightness around you, in which it is easier to move.

This is a fantastic detoxing exercise. We have seen people who perceptualize a heavy feeling and all kinds of grayish, blackish, and whitish stuff in their environment. When they do this exercise, the colors are transmuted, and their bodies feel as if made of a lighter material substance. The feeling of lightness is also a feeling of cleanliness. The blue cloud exercise can also detoxify you. Whenever people say that they see black, white, or gray, I know they are absorbing and throwing out, absorbing and throwing out. This is a good measuring stick for detoxing.

Another measuring stick for the changes that come with breathing exercises is your pulse. Take your pulse before and after each exercise. You are likely to find that after the exercise, your blood pressure has gone down. If you talk to any medical doctor, he or she will tell you that it is very easy to get blood pressure up, but it is very hard to get it down. We have seen people with hypertension experience a significant drop in blood pressure with these breathing exercises in minutes. This is a very good way of getting the pulse and the heart rate regulated in a good rhythm. It shows that your brain and breathing rhythm are starting to affect your body, and reveals to you your body's capabilities for self-regulation and self-healing.

Voluntary controls means to be able to have the conscious mind follow up in an appropriate way on what the unconscious directs it to do, so that it becomes a spontaneous expression. People often think control means that we can make things happen. But by voluntary controls, I mean learning to direct my awareness to what is on my horizon, so that my unconscious mind takes over and regulates my body without my having to think about it. The conscious thinking process constantly interferes with the development of voluntary controls. Holding on to thoughts, and living by society's belief systems instead of our own inner knowing, stops us from freeing our energy and from generating new energy. When we are thinking, doubting, questioning, or calculating, based on someone else's authority, we are operating in the beta brain wave state.

Beta is a high-frequency state, but it has a very low radiance—low energy output, very low voltage, very low amplitude. Your level of progressive excitement, your generative power, is also not very high. This is a state in which you are not very motivated to learn new information, because you think you already know it. In reality, you only have an outside knowledge of it; you do not have an inner experience of it.

To develop voluntary controls we cannot stay in this beta state. We must have our energy continuously active and operating in a generative capacity. We can only be affected negatively by outside events and the mental states of other people if we resonate with inappropriate environmental influences because we are operating inappropriately with our own energy. Just like you cannot take darkness into light, but you can take light into darkness, there is no way that lower energy, lower amplitude, lower voltage, low material energy can ever enter into high energy. The moment it hits that high energy, it is transformed into high energy.

Holding on to thoughts in the beta state ties up our energy in a molecular form in which it is affected by gravitation. When you wake up in the morning and have no interest in doing something exciting, you walk around like an elephant making dips in the floor. Everyone can not only feel you coming, they can hear you coming, too. If you weigh 150 pounds, you sound like you weigh 450. You have not gained weight but your energy is condensed in the matter of your body; the gravitational pull is very intense. You are really portraying that weight because you are not expanded.

Now, when you wake up in the morning enthusiastically, with a project on your mind that you are generative about, you float around like a butterfly. You make dips in the ceiling. You want to get out, and you still weigh 150 pounds. You float instead of going into the basement and making holes in the concrete. You have not physiologically changed per se, but you have, through your excitement, expanded your energy. You take up more space—subtle space.

We can use perceptualization to expand our energy, to create a higher state of excitement, a higher amplitude. In the early 1950s, I suddenly started to realize that at certain moments in my daily functioning, I would feel the need to get really high, but to stay anchored to my daily environment. I wanted to have my head in the clouds and my feet on the ground. I wanted to let my energy expand until I could pick up what was in the clouds, but could spread that energy out in a functional way on the earth. As I tried to find my way to this state, I found myself lifting my eyes and seemingly looking into my skull. I didn't consciously invent this as an exercise; it just happened. Then I would close my eyelids, and suddenly, there were all these flashes of light. I perceptualized just throwing the light out, and I started feeling as if I were floating, even though I was still very much down here.

Then, when I came to the United States, someone handed me a book called the *Aquarian Gospel of Jesus the*

Christ, written by Levi. In the fortieth chapter, it says that Jesus was in Persepolis, and he was going to train the magi of Persepolis to go into the temple of the brain. Jesus says, "Now put all your business problems aside; look deep into the temple of silence and there you will see the candle of the Lord all aflame. Then you will be able to perceive the ark in which are hidden the tablets of the past, present, and future." Wow, I thought, there is my exercise! There is what I am doing with my eyes. I am looking deep into the temple of my brain; I see the candle of the Lord all aflame. Suddenly, my consciousness expands and I know more about the past, present, and future.

A few years later I met some Tibetans. I learned that whenever they do their physiological feats, their magic, and their body control, they also do this exercise—the Tibetan eye roll. Later, I saw a Hindu guru do the same thing. I then realized that this was not such an uncommon exercise after all.

What happens during this exercise has to do with the field of spiraling energy that surrounds the body. As that energy field expands, it gets a higher voltage and becomes more and more subtle. It immediately embraces any environment you enter, so that, if you are prepared, nothing that anyone does against you can affect you. That is what we call "cosmic love."

At the posterior fontanel, cosmic energy enters the body. It hits the pineal gland, and goes through the energy centers along the spine—the cervicals, gonads, solar plexus, thymus, thyroid, pituitary, and pineal—which, through the ganglia, give energy to those organs. The pineal gland is not connected to the spine. But the pituitary gland, which is exactly above the spine, functions as a prism. The pituitary gland throws light down the spine; we call this the "speed train." The light hits the gonadic system—the root chakra, or sacrum. I call the sacral area my butane tank, with the pilot light on it. That is my fire. That is where the energy is densest, but very powerful.

I realized that in doing the Tibetan eye roll, you are looking at the light that comes from that prism. You may see as if looking through a tunnel, or through the barrel of a rifle. You might see it like a spiral. The moment that you start perceiving, or even feeling, that the light energy is coming to the forehead, immediately project that energy outward from the center of your forehead. This is the incoming energy going down, up, and out from the center of your forehead. That's why some statues have a jewel in the forehead. We have been able to measure electrically that this projected energy has a high output.

Throwing the light forward creates a cocoon of energy around you, which, as the output rises, becomes more subtle. More voltage builds up, your brain waves go into lower frequencies and higher amplitudes, and you go beyond the beta brain wave state. You also have greater immunity, because nothing of a lower energy can enter your energy field.

The Tibetans do the eye roll in a natural way. They do not do it deliberately as an exercise, but as something that happens spontaneously. I am sharing with you how I do it, but maybe you will find another way by which you can achieve the same results. I am not saying this is the only way. It has been used by many people, as well as by me, and seems to be a very good reprogramming procedure. Your eyes will show only white, but this is exactly what they do when they are connecting with your higher self. You don't need to feel that this is not normal or be frightened by it. We tend to misinterpret many things and hold ourselves back from being natural.

The first time you do this exercise, try it with your eyes open. It might hurt, because you have not used your eyes appropriately. Your eyelids are not just there to open and close your eyes; they are also for activating the retina. This activation is necessary to realize the energy held within the rods and cones. When the rods and cones are stimulated, releasing energy, they affect your chemistry through the optical nerve. They bring the light into your brain, activating the pyramidal cells. These become radiant, and the brain starts to operate properly with the eyelids.

Look at the ceiling for a moment. Ask yourself if you are looking up the way you normally would. Do it as you are used to; don't try to be good. Look to the side, now look to the other side; look at a spot on the floor. Are you using your eyes or your neck to turn to the side? Look up, look down, look left, look right, look around. If this is difficult, it is because muscles that need to activate the retina by motion have been stagnant, losing their elasticity, becoming sclerotic.

The average person perceives only about 10 percent of the light that enters his or her eyes; this 10 percent gets to the brain. The other 90 percent does not activate the brain because we do not use our eyes to look; we use our neck instead. What we call invisible can be made visible if we start using our eyes appropriately. This exercise by itself already helps you to start experiencing your energy field more perceptually than you ever have before. You also affect your entire brain and make it more functional. It is all interrelated. The more you do these exercises, the less pain you will have; you will overcome the sclerotic state and become more flexible. It is as if you had your arm in a cast and the cast were taken off; if you start moving it, it is going to hurt you. You are not going to stop moving your arm just because it hurts; you know that the hurt is healing. The same thing with your eyes.

The second step is to close your eyelids while your eyes stay rolled up. The eyes go up like a push-up, and the eyelids are pulled down, so you get a contradictory motion. Your eyelids may flutter a little. Keep your head up so that your spine is straight. Look deep into the back of your brain; you might see that light spot or light spots, or you might feel them; you might feel a kind of spaciness or a rise in temperature. Try to perceive that energy in the back—the light; either in feeling, seeing, or in some other way, perceptualize it. Look through a tunnel out of the center of your forehead; just keep projecting the light and keep your eyes closed. You can drop your eyes the moment you start projecting the light, but keep your eyelids closed.

The light that you see in the back of your head is coming through the pituitary gland, which functions as a prism, as a periscope reflecting the pilot light at the base of your spinal column. If you have spine curvature, you might not see it; you might only feel it. You are concentrating on the light within rather than the light from without. What you see is what you are projecting. This exercise helps you realize that your aura is only that which emanates from you, that radiates from you.

There is a relationship between brain wave states, perceptualization, and rapid eye movement (REM). I discovered this as part of the process I call the "cosmic review." In my books *Path of Action* and *Voluntary Controls*, I discuss how it can be helpful to take some time every night to review your experiences of the day and of the past. Once you have dealt with the past, this review becomes a daily maintenance that requires less and less time as you become more spontaneous. Where fifteen or twenty years ago it might have taken me an hour and a half to go over the day and look at everything from an appropriate and inappropriate point of view, now it takes me just seconds because I deal with the situation as it comes, when it comes, rather than storing it away in my subconscious mind. Now I spontaneously look for the solution and get away from the problem, rather than trying up the energy of my subconscious mind in old tapes in the filing cabinets. This makes the energy available for self-regulation.

Later, I discovered that REM could be used for the same purpose. Instead of mentally reviewing the details of my daily experience, I could immediately express them through perceptualization. When REM was first studied, it was believed to occur predominantly in the sleep state, but now we must realize we also do this when we are fully awake. Every time someone asks us a question, or we ask ourselves a question, our eyes make movements characteristic of one of the brain wave states.

Certain organizations have taken this as a way to do what they call "pacing" people. Thus, REM has a neurolinguistic aspect that tells us what is happening in the brain and, therefore, also in the body.

For example, suppose I ask you if you have read the *Aquarian Gospel of Jesus the Christ*. I might see your eyes go up first to the left and then go up to the right. The first movement is when you are trying to get the image of the book. The second movement is when you are trying to get the form of the words, and maybe some of the chapters or the title. Each direction the eyes move has a corresponding brain wave state.

Or I ask someone, "Have you been crying lately?" Immediately, her eyes look down to the left, not because she is shy, but because she is checking out her emotions. First, her eyes make a movement that indicates she is trying to get in touch with her emotions; and then her eyes move down and to the right as she tries to find the form of her emotions and see what they mean. Suppose I ask someone who likes music, "Do you remember the opera *La Traviata?*" His eyes move laterally—first to the left, where he tries to pick up the sound, and the combination of the sounds and words, or maybe even an image of the singers on stage. Eyes also move continually in response to other stimuli. For instance, if I smell something, the eyes go straight up. Now, let us have a piece of meat; the eyes go straight down. Straight up is smell; straight down is taste. Each of the five senses has a corresponding eye movement.

Suppose you ask people a question, and instead of REM, their eyes stay focused in the center. What do you think about them? Immediately you feel very comfortable with them because they are truthful to you.

When you ask them a question, they immediately give you a spontaneous answer, and their eyes stay focused. There is a man who once became a very public person, and we called him "Tricky," because whenever he talked, he could never keep his eyes in one position. He talked to you like this: "Well, ya, hum, hum"— he was constantly looking for answers in his emotions and in his memories. However, if your senses are synchronized and synthesized, your eyes stay focused in the center, and there is no REM.

We can use perceptualization to attain this voluntary control and direct our eye movements. Perceptualization involves the movement of the eyes in all directions, as we start to perceive with all our other senses and break the dependence on just our sense of vision. Many people, for instance, stop meditating because they think of it in terms of visualization, and they do not get anything but waves and colors, or they do not see any particular thing. They think, "I cannot visualize, so I won't meditate anymore; I won't try to imagine anything." Of course, if you see nothing when you mediate, you are seeing "nothing." It is a great blackness, but you are still activating your sense of vision; your eyes are moving. We can use these REM to activate all the senses and eventually to synthesize them.

Now, a lot of people perceptualize inside their heads rather than outside. To me, this is too crowded already. I want to be free, in the open, so I create a horizon and put my images on it. By images, I do not necessarily mean I give them form. I allow the unconscious to give them form if that is necessary. A wave can be a form; it does not need to be a specific, recognizable shape or object.

Here is an exercise using perceptualization and eye movement. First establish your horizon. For a moment let yourself feel, sense, perceptualize outside, on your horizon. You can do this with your eyes closed or open, but it is best with your eyes closed, so that you do not get distracted by things around you. Try to put your horizon as far away from you as possible.

Now, imagine that the sun has just come above the horizon. Imagine a huge disk there, and then allow the disk to become a clock dial. See the numbers twelve, one, and so on. Now, imagine you wind up the clock and move your eyes clockwise around the dial, starting at 11 o'clock. This corresponds to the upward-to-the-left REM. Now go to 12 o'clock; this is the eye position that activates your sense of smell. Then go to 1 o'clock, which activates the forming of words and images. At 3 o'clock is one of the lateral REM; at 5 o'clock, the activation of emotions; at 6 o'clock, your sense of taste is activated. Continuing on, 7 o'clock is again your emotions, 9 o'clock again your lateral REM; and then, you are back at 11 o'clock. Make sure you do indeed move your eyes around your imaginary clock dial. Now, go around again a little faster. Stop for a moment; then do it counterclockwise, slowly at first and then a little faster. Stop again. Open your eyes and just let it fade out.

This exercise is very good for straightening out the filing cabinets of your subconscious mind without needing to rely on concepts or searching for the meaning of your sense images. Instead, you are free to perceptualize, and you might find as you do this exercise that you have many different sense perceptions. This is also a good exercise to do for a few seconds before you do other perceptualizations.

Here is another way to look at why it is good to go beyond a concern for the meaning of sense images. Some of you may have been taught to meditate by concentrating on geometrical figures on your horizon. You may have been told to make sure that you did not lose your image. Every time you lost your image, you were supposed to set it up again. However, when I meditate, I am a fisherman and the universal mind is the pond or ocean where I go fishing. Whatever I consciously put as an image on my horizon is my bait. It would be silly, when the cosmos finally nibbles, for me to try to put my bait back again. If my image disappears, I know that the universe is biting. I let it bite, and a new image comes up. I am not interested in the meaning of that new image. I just use it as my bait. If I catch a dolphin, I throw the dolphin back at my horizon. Again I get a nibbling, and it might be a whale or a whole school of dolphins.

The act of the sense perception is more important to me than the meanings of many of the images that come up. The motion is actually straightening out your energy fields, which is much more important than any understanding of a particular sense image. Later on, if you have done this often enough, you can go into a dream state and have lucid dreams in which the so-called interpretation will automatically come. You will know intuitively what you have picked up and what the meaning is for you—and not the meaning according to this or that book, or this or that teacher; you will have your own interpretation of your sense images.

Another exercise I often use is one in which you can perceptualize the interior of your body to diagnose what is going on in there. The first part of the exercise is to become more aware of your sense perception, to become hyperaesthetic, hypersensitive. The second part is to imagine traveling through your body with that heightened sense perception, using your energy to perceive, observe, and restore in a nonjudgmental way by beaming light on whatever you find. To begin, go into a relaxed state by doing your breathing exercises to regulate your body. Start with alpha breathing—inhale for eight counts, hold in for eight, hold out for four. Do this three times. Then go to theta breathing in order to get in touch with the intuitive mind. Inhale for four counts, hold in for eight, exhale for sixteen, hold out for four. Do this once or twice. Now go into your meditative state by closing your eyes and setting up your horizon. Perceive on your horizon a mirror image of your physical self. Knowing that you are still sitting in your room, observe through your senses your mirror image. You may use your sense of vision, or you may only feel yourself there as a tactile perception. Start by using your sense of touch and feeling the form on the horizon. Feel the parts of the form on your body. Feel your face, nose, skull, neck, and shoulders as they occur on your horizon. Feel your chest, back, abdomen, trunk, thighs, calves, ankles, and feet. Feel the ground you are standing on and the air surrounding you.

Now, focus on your sense of smell. Smell all aspects of your environment and your own being, and become aware of the new images, the different fragrances. There might be something in the environment that you become sensitive to, which you were not paying attention to before. This can enhance your sense perception by making you aware of the things that are surrounding you and how they relate to your own senses.

Now, switch to the sense of taste. Taste your environment and your own being. Notice how certain feelings and aspects of your experience create different tastes. Identify them without labeling them. Just become aware of them by heightening your sense perception.

Now, start to hear all the sounds in your environment. Become sensitive to the sounds you bring forth, which might be occurring below or beyond the normal audible level. Become aware that by expanding your consciousness, expanding your energy, you become more sensitive to the sounds of your body. Make that which was seemingly inaudible become audible for you. In a non-attached way, register whatever sounds are occurring in the environment, and what other sounds are coming forth from you, and how they integrate together.

Finally, use your sense of vision to perceive what you can bring forth of the form that represents you on the horizon, and experience the energy as it comes forth from you. Gaze alongside the image of yourself. Become aware of particular objects, substances, forms, or energy fields in the environment surrounding you. Become aware of particular colors as the different frequencies of the energy radiate at you and from you. Make an effort to get a good visual image of that form of yourself on the horizon.

Having awakened all your sense perceptions and brought them to a heightened state, and having expanded your awareness of self and what you represent in your environment physically, mentally, and spiritually, continue with this meditation by using your imagination to take the energy from you sitting in your room and direct it at your image on your horizon of self. It does not have to be exactly a mirror image any longer, but any image as it comes from you on the horizon. Allow it to be there and direct your energy toward it, as if you were projecting laser beam energy at that particular image of self on your horizon. While you are projecting your energy, imagine that you perceive your image—feel it, see it, hear it, taste it, smell it—growing to a very big size. And while it is growing, feel your own physical beingness and image, as it sits in your room, becoming microscopically small in comparison with the image on your horizon.

On that image on your horizon, find any of its openings, any of its orifices—the eyes, ears, nostrils, pores, genital area, rectum. Find any opening and allow the microscopically small image of your physical self to be projected into the huge image of self. Enter that image and travel through it as if it were a giant statue. Observe without making changes. Register what it feels like, what it sounds like, what it looks like, what it tastes like.

If you reach a place where you feel stagnant, just release a beam of energy from your forehead like a laser beam. Throw light on it and move on. Just observe and register what you are observing for later recall. Your mind is responsive to this and will register every perception you have. Whether or not this eventually comes to your conscious mind, it is within your unconscious, experienced and registered. So travel wherever you want. Stop and observe a little closer whenever you want. You are in command. Just keep projecting your light wherever you move through that giant image of self.

Now find an exit. It might be the same place you entered, or you might be closer to another exit. At whatever place you feel you can exit as a microscopically small being, move out of the giant statue. Allow the microscopic image of self to blend again with your physical self, to reenter into the physical self and become one with it.

Observe the giant statue as it takes its normal size again. Observe it for a couple of seconds and notice if any changes are observable to you through your senses. Now, take a deep abdominal breath, inhale and exhale. Once more, take a very deep inhalation, release it with a sigh, and let go. Once more inhale deeply, and let go. Now inhale and exhale abdominally several times. Whenever you feel ready, open your eyes.

I have done this inner body perceptualization exercise with many young children, under seven years of age, who have absolutely no anatomical background. Instead of asking for verbal feedback, we asked them to draw what they had experienced during this trip through the image of their body. Quite often, these children drew pictures of organs that were anatomically correct, practically right out of a textbook. We knew then that they had really experienced their bodies and had been able to perceptualize their organs.

In a recent session of our children's course at the Aletheia Center, a boy perceptualized going into his finger, which he had damaged a little while before. He found a little piece missing in one of the little finger bones, and went searching for it. He found it and brought it back to where it was missing. Before this exercise he did not have enough power in his hands to pull himself up in gymnastics. After this particular session, he was immediately able to use his hands to hang from an exercise bar.

I am sharing this with you to help you understand that these states of so-called fantasy have a lot of value. Your unconscious really knows how you look on the inside, so you can actually use perceptualization as a diagnostic tool, to go into your body and check it out. Sometimes people climb their spines and discover all kinds of things. People go to the stomach or become aware of other organs. Some go through the blood vessels and find, "Gee, there is some stuff on the inner walls." They laser beam it, and it starts to break off nicely in their perceptualization. There is no way to predict what will happen. Each person will have his own individual experience.

Do not, however, make any conscious decision to

change. You can make changes only by throwing light on the problem. The light is high energy. If your body needs to be healed, it will be changed, without your deciding, "Aha, this should look like this or that; it should operate this way or that way; I'll do something about it." Rather than using the thinking process or logic, just flood it with your light, and whatever needs to be done will be done. The healing will take place if something needs to be healed.

Again, however, do not judge yourself. It is not necessary to see anything. Even if you just sense a form to be there, that is enough. You may find that you just have a nonvisual sense of doing the entire exercise. You may imagine you enter a pore of the form you project onto your horizon without ever seeing it.

There is no need to compare your experience to anyone else's. Suppose someone tells you he could visualize the form of his body very clearly, the whole body, and it becomes like a beautiful model, a translucent image of a Greek god, and he went into his ear and traveled through the body. But you only perceived a tiny hole, with a little bit of orange, a little bit of purple, and a little bit of pink. You may think, "We have a master here who got it, and I am not even a beginner in comparison." It is not necessary to feel that way.

Other people's experience, including mine, can only give you a map. You have to walk the territory, and what you find does not necessarily have to be as the map says. Start to listen to your own inner authority and your own experience. Then you can help others draw their maps. Sometimes in groups I find it tough even to ask for feedback, because the students quite often try to outdo each other, and not necessarily consciously. But I have seen people stop doing exercises because they felt they were not able to do them as well as others.

Be good to yourself and perceive how it feels. That is the most important thing—how did it feel when you went through the exercise? Did it feel good? Did you get a little irritated because you did not get what you wanted? When I guide people through a perceptualization, sometimes their obedience to me disturbs their experience; they try to do something that doesn't work for them. As your guide, I only temporarily function as your ground control; *you* are flying your rocket. I can sit here and look on my screen and say, "Well, this is what she should do; it is better for her," but you are the one experiencing it. You have to make the decision about what to do. I am only guiding you. This is why we suggest that you put these exercises on tape, with pauses between each sentence, so that your own voice guides you.

Suppose you are doing this exercise, and halfway through you lose track of the guide and you are on your own. You may hear your tape in the distance, but you are doing other things. It is marvelous if you go off on your own because it makes the experience even richer. You are learning disobedience to outer authority, and obedience to inner authority—your own authority, your own knowingness. All the while, of course, your unconscious is still registering the voice of your guide, and if you need to, you can always fall back on my map.

This is how you learn to start trusting your own perceptions, so that even if a guide is there, you know how to use perceptualization to get into that mediation state. You have to learn to trust yourself. Once you have gotten to know your own territory, you won't need my map anymore.

Most people who first do this exercise flip back and forth between alpha and theta brain wave states. It is as if you are still checking—"Do I have everything with me? Do I have my insurance policies? Will I still know how to come back?" This happens not in thoughts, but in feelings.

Another experience you may have is the feeling that in the middle of the exercise you have drifted off and fallen asleep. What happens is that you are in mind/body harmony state, associated with theta or delta brain waves. You may feel as if it is a sleep state, but at the end of the exercise you come back to normal consciousness much more easily than you would if you were really asleep. So it is not sleep. It is a state in which you are in a more outwardly expanded state of consciousness. You still have control here, but you are, at the same time, over there, and you do not pay attention anymore. You know how you might be talking to one person, looking straight at them, and, therefore, seemingly not paying any attention to someone else. But if that other person moves, you can still perceive that movement on the periphery of your vision. It is the same thing with your not hearing the voice of your guide anymore, or hearing it as a hum and not getting the words. You are starting to go into expanded consciousness. Your attention moves away from the guiding voice, and you go on your own guidance—which is good.

You may wonder why you had the exact experience you did during the exercise and how it affects you personally. Every experience has its value, you do not need to judge. A relaxed feeling is similar to the mind/body harmony that takes place in the theta and delta wave states. A sense of expanded feeling that slows you down should remind you of how, with a greater momentum, time itself slows down. Frequently, you cannot tell how long your session has lasted. If you did not get lucid perceptions, then you know that you were working on being in tune with other aspects of the universe. So, if you ask "Why did I do that?" it is not *why* did you do it but *what* did you do that is important. What was the effect of it, while your body was relaxed and not interfering with your perception level?

Some people find it a little hard to think immediately after the exercise. This does not mean you are not thinking, but that you are not as affected by all the thoughts coming in. Your mind is in a much more flowing state. There are still a lot of things coming in at once, but now they are all nicely integrated and synthesized, and your energy is much more stable. You are more harmonious, inside and out, less stressed. There is no fight with the outer environment; there is a flowing with it.

There is one more exercise I would like to share with you, which also deals with perceptualization. This exercise, called the "Seven Doors" exercise, is found in the book *Voluntary Controls*. You can put this on tape to guide you through it, but, remember, you are on your own.

Get yourself in a relaxed state. Take a couple of deep breaths—abdominal, diaphragmatic—and really feel your body sitting wherever you are. Become aware of the room that you are in. Now perceive your horizon. Put your attention away from the here and now as if you were looking at the curvature of the horizon, where you normally would see the sun rise. See the sky, and allow the perception to become clear. Between where you are sitting and your horizon there is a beautiful, grassy meadow running from you all the way to the horizon; it is lush and green.

Now between you and the horizon allow yourself to perceive a second image of yourself. It does not have to be a mirror image, just an image that comes forth from your creation of your inner being. Become the guide for this second image; direct it to move over the meadow, to experience the coolness of the grass, the blueness of the sky, the warmth of the sun, the smell of flowers, the rushing of the water in the distance. Guide the image to move toward the horizon, until close to horizon it reaches a knoll.

Looking down from the knoll, allow your second image to discover a three-story building, slightly down the slope. Direct your second image to go and explore this building, to move around it and observe it, and find that it has two doors that open up like French doors, and three little steps down. Direct your second image to go down the three steps and be confronted by a long corridor. On the left there are seven doors, each a specific color. Observe these doors and the colors of the doors without trying to name the colors. Allow your second image to move spontaneously through this corridor and to choose a door on the left, and observe it. The door might have some statement written on it, identifying what lies beyond it, or it might just be a blank door with a specific color.

Allow your second image to open that door and

to go through it into the space you find there. Explore that space, whatever your unconscious shows it to be. Should it be dark, then shine light on it. Should it be light, resonate with it. Observe it, relate to it, interact with it if you so choose. Observe any changes taking place within that space and within your second image.

Now, withdraw your second image outside of that space beyond the door, back into the corridor again, and allow the door to stay ajar behind you. Let your unconscious second self determine which door, which space, on the right side of the corridor it wants to explore. Observe the color or statement on the chosen door. Open the door and go through it. Perceive what is occurring there, and, again, if you so desire, interact, or just be an observer. Allow your unconscious to register all your second image experiences there. When you feel your task is fulfilled, allow your second image to exit this space, and again leave the door ajar behind you.

Move toward what seems to be the end of this corridor. Just when you have nearly reached the end, discover that it is transparent, yet reflective, like a mirror. But it is not of substance; it is an energy field. Observe your second self while encountering this energy field at the end of the corridor. Can you perceive any changes taking place? You are all-powerful and all-energy, which can increase in power and in its ability to penetrate. Allow your second image to penetrate this mirrorlike energy field. Move through it to find yourself entering into a round space, like a round room without a ceiling, but with a floor of claylike substance. Perceive your second self moving to the center of this circular space. Try to remember any feelings you may get somewhere in this circular space.

Hidden just a few inches underneath the soft surface of the clay is an ancient book. Find your second self moving to where your unconscious knows this ancient book, open it up and page through it dispassionately. Observe what each page might represent. Check out your feeling level, while paging through this book. Since you have at least become acquainted with the book and some of what you might have observed to be on the pages, put it back where you found it. At any given time in the future you can always go back to this space and find the book and explore it further. After you have buried the book in the clay, notice whether you are facing north, northeast, or northwest; south, southwest, or southeast; or just west or east. Remember this.

Go back to the center of this circular space without ceilings, but with an adobe floor. Somewhere in this room, also underneath the soil, in a different direction or the same direction, there is another hidden book. It is also just a few inches down, if at all, buried in the clay. Go and find it and dig it out. Observe it. Page through it and find it to be quite a new book,

not ancient like the other one. Again, for later rec-
ollection, close the book, and put it back and note
where you put it, so at a later date you can always go
back and explore it further if you so desire. Your unconscious registers where your book is hidden.

Now bring your second self back to the center
again, and move toward that energy field through
which you entered into this circular space. Exit the
room, moving again through that energy field. Observe if it feels any different from when you entered.
Now find your second self in the corridor again, with
the seven doors on the left and the seven doors on the
right. Of course, what was left is now right, it is
reversed. Once more, turn around and perceive. Gaze
into the mirrorlike energy field at the end of the corridor. Perceive and register any changes that have
taken place.

As soon as you feel up to it, move through the
corridor toward the three steps. As you go, observe if
the doors you left ajar are still open. Climb the three
steps and open the double French doors again, and
find your second self back in the green meadow on
the knoll.

Observe yourself sitting on the chair in this room.
Allow your second image to move over the meadow
toward you on the chair, and to reenter, to reintegrate
with your physical being. Let this be a gentle action.
Take a very deep breath and let go with a sigh. Once

more, take a deep inhalation, and let go with a sigh; take a deep inhalation, and let go with a sigh. Now inhale and exhale, faster, and just let go. Whenever you feel up to it, open your eyes.

This exercise combines fantasies, reveries, and guided dreams in such a way that they deal with your emotional, mental, physical, and spiritual aspects. We can do any type of fantasy, but sometimes we just do a fantasy for fantasy's sake. That three-story house, of course, and the meadow, I put up there as symbols of growth in your beingness, your body. The corridor with the seven doors is a symbol of your spinal canal with the seven chakras; the ones on the left are your feminine sides, the ones on the right your masculine. For instance, the third door on the left, from the bottom up, symbolizes the solar plexus chakra. If you found the door to be, let us say, gold instead of green (the color of the chakra), then you know that there was a predominant aspect of your consciousness directed to your emotional plane on your feminine side. You can use this exercise as a diagnostic tool if you do not put anything consciously, purposely in there, but allow it all to happen. Again, my guidance can be a map, but let your unconscious create your experiences. Notice how I asked you to go into the *space* beyond the door. I am very careful when I identify these places that I do not suggest an image that holds you back from further exploration. I did not say a house, because some of you might not have perceived a house; you might have imagined a temple or a castle, a tower, or whatever.

The energy field at the end of the corridor represents your inner transition from the personal to the transpersonal. That is why I ask you first to look into the energy field as a reflecting mirror. Then you can go into that rounded room, which represents the universal beingness; you go beyond your body to the transpersonal self. The ancient book buried in the adobe floor represents your past life, whatever it may have been. The new book represents your future life.

Do not interpret these symbols literally, but rather go by the feelings you got from the experience. Remember that anytime you wish, you can go back to that place.

For some people, the first book represents hidden knowledge, and they are afraid to read it. There is no reason to be afraid. This symbol comes from your unconscious mind, and if you are really not supposed to have some forbidden knowledge, your unconscious would not show it to you. It is only forbidden until it is shown to you. There is very little sense in teasing you with something that is forbidden. The future book will let you know what to do with it.

One person who did this exercise told me afterward as she began to go out on her horizon, she just let herself go. She saw her second self passing the solar system and looking up at the celestial dome. Then she heard me say, "Now be in a meadow," and she thought, "I've got to go back." She immediately dropped all that she was imagining, came back, and restructured her vision. This is exactly what I would suggest to you *not* to do. You should be obedient only to your own unconscious, not to any guide or teacher. Once you are already discovering your own horizons and farther places, why go back to what the teacher says? Perhaps you are afraid you will lose your guide. Well, even if you do, you can either think, "Gee, I lost him," or, "Thank God I lost him!" It all depends on whether or not you are secure in what you are experiencing yourself, and are glad you do not need someone else's map.

Sometime you may have been traveling by car and thought you were lost, even though you might have been there before. You stop at the service station and buy a map. But the moment you take the map in your hands, you remember where you are going, without looking at the map. You put the map in your glove compartment, and you find the place on your own. You don't need the map, but it gives you a feeling of security. The structure I give is for those who are not yet on their way. For those of you who have gone beyond the map, please do not make yourself come back.

7

SEX,
POWER,
AND MONEY

It's easy to be misunderstood when we talk about sex, power, and money. They sound so unspiritual. But integrated, they are only another form of body, mind, and spirit—or matter, mind, and spirit—the foundations of the universe. We tend to forget that we live in a very sexual universe that would not exist without energy in a state of motion, continuously transforming and being transformed through creative acts. Creation is not something that happened once at the beginning of time. It is not something that uses up energy. I like to say that God never gave up creating; He didn't retire. And He wasn't tired the first time.

Sex, power, and money all have to do with the universal energy that not only transforms continuously, but also maintains the perfect organization and harmony of the universe. They are like the three pillars that support the capital of a Greek temple. They are our economic capital, too—the source of all our other forms of energy.

The universal energy is always either positive or negative, but these are terms we often misunderstand. We are not talking about good and bad. We tend to use positive to mean good. But suppose you have had a biopsy, and the doctor calls you up and says the test is positive. Suddenly positive is very bad. Does that mean if you tell me to have positive thoughts, I should be bad? And if the doctor says the test is negative, you get champagne; you celebrate. Suddenly negative is good.

We must realize that positive only means energy with a positive electrical charge, and negative means negatively charged energy. But these states of electrical charge have definite qualities. Positive is masculine and negative is feminine. Positive energy is always contracting, and negative energy is always expanding. Positive energy goes from the outside to the center, and negative energy goes from the center to the outside.

Positive goes clockwise, negative goes counterclockwise. As we see with pendulums and light, positive energy is centripetal and negative energy is centrifugal. In the Orient, the masculine positive is yang, the feminine negative yin.

In wave/line theory, when the positive and negative converge with each other, become harmonious and neutral, they create a current. When they separate again, there is a burst of energy that peaks in amplitude, up and down, continuously spiraling.

Our bodies also operate on these principles of positive and negative, feminine and masculine. It just so happens that most men have a slightly higher—maybe a half percent—positive, or masculine, charge, and women a slightly higher negative, or feminine, charge. The negative is more emotional and more expandable than the positive, which is more contracted. So, masculine and feminine are not a matter of gender, but of positive and negative electro-potentials.

These two states of energy must continuously have union with each other, maintaining the universe in a neverending cocreative act. The electrical potential of the positive and negative, the masculine and feminine, must continuously have sex. My standard joke is, Why are you so against sex? Because if my potassium stops having sex with my sodium, my whole nervous system goes kaput.

Sex is actually the activity of our capital. Unless

that energy has sex we have no solvency. Many people have a lot of possessions, but they are not solvent. They look for results, but once the result is achieved, what else is there to do? They try to maintain a balance, but balance can become very static. What is needed is a balance that immediately releases itself so that it can go into a state of transformation to find harmony and balance again. It is not a static result, but a process. It is energy maintaining an ever-changing harmony, continuously having sex.

In the past we have looked upon sexuality only as a means of physical gratification or procreation, rather than as a cocreative act of energy transformation. We now have trouble recognizing the feminine aspect. We have been result- and orgasm-oriented, and this has been the basis for our entire political and economic state, though we call it by different names. This orientation has affected every aspect of our lives, from our relationships to our health to the way we understand nuclear energy. In politics, in fact, we are fission-oriented. Interestingly enough, orgasm and fission are the same thing.

In biochemistry we talk about the continuous harmonizing of acid-forming substances and base-forming substances. Here is an image of transformation and harmony: physical substances are released out then made solvent again. Acid forming is the solvent, making the substance solvent again, releasing the energy out of its material base-forming state. None of us are good with just bases. We need to go beyond.

Every creative act we do beyond procreation is to maintain our spaces. Nature takes care of this in its spiritual way, doing things we don't understand with our so-called logical thinking. For instance, some forest fires occur naturally, started by lightning. We fight these fires. But the trees that are full grown will only be slightly scorched, and the underbrush which was actually smothering all the saplings and making it impossible for wild life to find food will be burned away. Spaces are maintained.

Earlier in this book I discussed how energy coming into the body hits the pineal gland, in ancient times called the third eye, and the pituitary gland. Now we have discovered that the proteins in our retina are the same proteins found in our pineal gland, so that we can speak about the retinal factor of the pineal gland. But the pineal and pituitary glands are also gonadotropic. That is, they also activate the generative process—your gonads. In the female these are the ovaries and the uterus, and in the male the testes and the prostate.

What do you generate? The same energy exchanges as throughout the universe. What takes place in the universe is a spiritual union of the masculine positive and the feminine negative particles, the sexual act. In the physiological, biological state it is the spiritual union of the positive and negative, the masculine and the feminine, within your own body. In every act you do, whether it is being intimate with someone special or tying your shoes, you need to generate this sexual activity.

I will never forget the day that I was in Claremont, California, in a Lutheran church as a visiting minister. I had given my sermon, and then there was a question period. One person asked, "What about sex?" I looked over the congregation, and suddenly I said, "I want to have intercourse twenty-four hours a day." Well, after the mushroom cloud had died down, I explained that what I meant was that I wanted to have intercourse with God. For if God is present in all things, then I need to interact, interrelate with everything. I have to be radiant. And if I have no lust, I will not shine, all my energy will be kept inside, in my butane tank, with even my pilot light turned down.

In everything you do, everything you desire to express, to be cocreative you need to activate your gonadic system. You have to get the spark. Incitement is not enough. You know what happens when we incite the population: we get riots, and we have to call in the riot squad. You have a riot squad, too: your spleen. If your ignition system doesn't work and the generator blows off, for whatever reason, and you have no energy left, you can immediately send in your National Guard, your reserves, to take care of it.

I have met people who claim to be spiritual, yet they live from the neck up. The lower part of their bodies are not important anymore. I never understand how they can do it. How can you get light and energy up in the attic without going down to the basement and turning the pilot light up or the fuse box on? Every action we do involves intercourse—charge and discharge. What needs to be excited in order to do any creative act? You need to excite that engine in your attic called the brain. In every act you do, you must have a personal intercourse, a spiritual union of your feminine and masculine aspects. Sexuality must go beyond orgasm, which is the big boom only in the lower part of your body. When the positive and the negative come together, they blend, they integrate spiritually, unadulterated, without any ulterior motivations. Motive, to have spiritual union, raises the energy and fuses it within what we call the heart. This has to do with the thymus gland, your immune system, and your seed of consciousness.

So you actually, within your own body, bring your feminine and masculine particles together, and a current is created. A current for what? A current you bring out to express. When we say that every act is a spiritual act, we mean that the soul is the essence. The energy is drawn out of our spiritual capital. You must have interest when you are putting something in your capital. If you have no interest, you are not going to be interested. You are not going to be incited; therefore, you are not going to be excited. We can use these words of economics to help us understand energy exchanges in every part of our lives.

The positive and the negative energies become a current streaming through you from your butane tank. They go up to the top and are expressed through motivation, through the "I will," which then fulfills "Thy will." The energies must be fused to come out in harmony. You create for cocreation by becoming as radiant as possible. That is your discharge.

Sitting in meditation is fine if you want to become passive. People sit and charge, and charge, and charge. They are like batteries. Then they come out of meditation never discharging, and they are surprised when their batteries start to leak. They need to do something creative, because that completes the whole process. We often use power to overpower people, rather than to activate ourselves. But put (e)nergy and (m)otion together, with power behind it, and we (em)power people. We empower people wherever we radiate.

I can say I am having sex with all of you reading this book—except perhaps those of you who have closed yourselves off. There is an exchange taking place, a harmonious motion, creating a world filled with light and the potential for healing.

Allow your energy to go out. Don't hold it back, don't be embarrassed about it. Have some lust in your life. A person without lust has no luster, and is listless. There is no radiance coming from that person. A person who is not healthy is also not going to be very sexy.

I call myself "Hot Pants Jack." I keep that generator going the whole day, and I do not turn it off even at night. During the two hours I sleep, I make sure that engine keeps running. You can never tell.

To follow a spiritual path, some people remain celibate, but that does not mean they are not having sex. They are abstaining from sexual intercourse, but they are having sex within themselves and using that energy. The men still actually use semen. The women use a form of seminal fluid also. Celibates go through an orgasm, but instead of directing it out from the bottom, they bring it all the way up where it hits the pituitary gland and affects all the chemistry in the brain. They are in a state called euphoria, a contained ecstasy. They become healthier and more radiant.

The writing of a beautiful poem can be a sexual, cocreative act that puts the masculine and the feminine together. It must contract to get form, then expand to discharge energy, and then contract into a new form, again and again until the poem is complete. Using your creative power requires that both hemispheres of your brain integrate that energy and interrelate with your body. What incites must also be regulated in turn. Your metabolism is activated before you start to express with your thyroid. As your thyroid gets more activated, it also becomes more balanced, and your metabolism is nicely regulated. Then you are ready and able to create outside of yourself. And when the "I will" becomes "Thy will be done," you affect the pure light that you are charging and discharging.

Money is part of that. When we bring the soul and the mind together, we get a current that stimulates the transformation of the material form by which we then maintain our physiological health. The soul is the source, the mind the director, and the body the material form in which the process of energy transformation, charge and discharge, takes place. Therefore, every act of soul, mind, and body is a sexual act that is also a spiritual act. The faster you charge and discharge, with desire and excitement, the less you stagnate, and the healthier you are.

Isn't this exactly how we understand the laws of economics? Your transformation, charges and discharges, goes beyond only expression and becomes an exchange. I like to say, if you want to change, you get change. And to have change you must have the process of exchange—exchange between you and the universe. You enhance everyone in your environment by discharging, and that becomes your currency. You start with your capital, and if you are interested, you will get interest. Through continuous sexual and spir-

itual energy exchange, you make your material substance solvent again.

When we talk about prosperity, the richness lies
within our spiritual aspects. There is no reason why
you cannot have everything in abundance—if you
keep exchanging, if you keep giving. Do you realize
that we have about 500,000 thoughts per second going
through our brains? And do you realize most of them
are old ones? Then you ask yourself, "Why don't I see
any changes in me?" Changes need to be stimulated.
You must have the desire, and desire cannot come
unless you have sexuality, unless you activate your
gonadic system and become aroused. Get the excitement and bring the desire all the way up until it becomes a transformational charge of knowing, of
healing. Then you must express it, discharge it, share
it, become part of energy exchanged.

Many of you say, "My cup runneth over." But do
you know where it is running to? Many roads can be
destroyed by cups that are running over. If you cannot
express why your cup runs over and share it with other
people, then you are not worthy of that abundance.
With every new thought you create, you cocreate with
God, the universe, and the spiritual power. You cocreate new conditions not just for yourself, but for
everyone who ever comes into your environment. You
see, you cannot stop your light. Your abundance is

infinite; the more you can get, the more you can give.

Right now in our world, sex, power, and money are the three biggest topics of control. Yet, for all the attention paid to them, we lack the understanding that they are energies that are there for us to use appropriately. In the Scriptures, particularly in the Old Testament, every sentence seems to mention "begetting" at least three times. What does begetting mean? It means being and getting, getting and giving—giving birth, not just to children, but giving birth to anything that needs to be materialized in this world to fulfill the function of the universe. In order to beget, we have to become. *Become* contains a sexual pun on orgasm—did you come already?—which reminds us to ask the next question: Are we going to beget, and do something with it? Or are we just going to sit in awe of sex and let the big bang go without using that energy? That would be spending a lot of time and effort and money on just a couple of kicks, wouldn't it? It would be like spending a lot of money on fireworks, which lose their creative power once you've shot them into the air.

We must realize that sexuality can also be used to create abundance. We have to give. We must let go and not look for results, and instead we must dare to have intercourse with the future. Whatever you're after, you're going to get.

When you think about abundance and prosperity,

don't look at amounts; don't look at forms. Look at the process. And don't limit the process, because if you do, you will limit that which needs to come forth from it. In thinking about money, it is very important to empower yourself by trusting the universe and putting out what you really want.

What's my motivation for building a health campus with so many acres, with buildings here and buildings there? I want people to come out of the Center healthy, brazen with radiance, empowered, ready to help the rest of the world find the integrity of that wave force. I want to help create a healthy world, a harmonious world, in which we know how to use sex, power, and money. The Center is a tool that helps make the process work. Do you think God doesn't listen? That God doesn't know? God is all-knowing and, therefore, you are, too—if you would just pay a little attention.

Every time in my life when it seemed I would receive no help, bang, it came through. You do not go after it. Instead, you must understand the flow of energy going through you. And you have to be willing to give.

The more you give, the more you receive, as long as you do not give in order to receive. Because if you give for that reason, it does not work. Your motivation is very important. For instance, many of us have thought that by giving some money to the poor, or giving money to a person who is in need, we are helping them, but quite often we are not. If your motivation in giving them a dollar is to get them away, it is not going to work for you either. The more you are able to recognize that you have to be excited, that you must have desire to reach out into the universe, the more you will connect and be able to exchange energy by putting it into material form. If that form happens to be money, then it is money. Your prosperity, however, is not measured by the amount of money you have, but by your capacity to be able to exchange, share, be, and become. That is where your abundance will lie. But you have to free yourself, trust that it is there, and set your process to work.

Help your fellow man by getting into a state of harmony yourself, by having a better understanding of the sexes, and by empowering other people. How can you do that? By shining your light and embracing them with your beingness. Then there will be an exchange. The moment you give, you will get—and get in abundance. It does not make any difference in what material form. It is going to be there.

It is so sad for me to see our lack of understanding for each other, the lack of exchange. We need to have sex within ourselves all the time, yet we mistake gender for sex and get absolutely frightened by it. We men have to work as hard to get our femininity out as women have to work to bring their masculinity out and develop their capacities to have the power to live in this world in equality. A lot of women are now doing masculine work. That does not necessarily mean man's work, but work that is contracting energy and masculine in form. My wife oversees our whole organization and takes care of all the financial aspects. If it were up to her, if she wrote a letter to the president of IBM because her computer was not working, she would say, "Dear John, while I'm watching the butterfly against my window, I hear the whisper of the autumn leaves rippling down, and I see the first fall storms coming up in the distance around the mountains. I would like you to know that my computer does not work anymore." She could be very dramatic, romantic, and spontaneous—very feminine, emotional, and energy expansive. Instead, she has to say, "Hey John, if I can call you that, I paid 10,000 dollars for this computer system and it still does not work."

When women go out into the work world, they are already uniformed for it. They all wear nice tailored business suits and carry an attaché case—masculine contracting energy. And when they come home, they are out of balance, because they have had to use all their masculinity and were not capable of putting their feminine, intuitive, spontaneous, romantic, and emotional qualities to work. What could they do about it? They could get into a colorful long robe, dance a little, listen to music, and meditate, rather than fix a double martini. They want to make themselves expansive.

We can see that under a conservative business regime there is very little freedom. Do you realize how much hypertension, how much excess stress is because of our misunderstanding of sex, power, and money? You do not need to be confused. You can use your power to empower. You can have sex without touching anyone. You can interrelate to others through your light, your radiance, the source and vehicle of all information. Nonverbal communications are very important, but so-called chemical attraction is still physical, material, the lowest most contracted form of the pure energy of your being. We need to release our energy from its contracted forms, from the masculine aspect. We need to relate in order to expand and to become creative again, to make our energy solvent again.

When you give, you will receive. Remember your true motivation, and make it a part of your beingness. In my giving to you, I have a tremendous joy, so I have already received the joy. Joy comes from the process, because my motivation is to love you forever. The receiving is there already, so I do not need to have expectations. I have something else, an expectancy, an inner knowing that I am getting something back. You can learn to trust your inner being and let out your radiance. Then sex, power, and money are yours for the giving.

8

RADIANT
HEALTH

"And God said, 'Let there be light,' and there was light!" This means that there will always be light, because light can never cease to be. Even darkness is not the absence of light, but the absorption of light. The radiant energy of the light is still there.

When you were created, you, too, were part of that light. That's why you enter the world—to be and to take part of the excitement of universal beingness. Then you see and hear the tall adults leaning over you, saying: "We have a son." "We have a daughter." "Now we have a bassinet." "We have a nursery prepared." Then the relatives come to look: "Oh, she has such a nice cute face." "He has his father's feet." They talk so much about what you have that you start putting together the two words *be* and *have* and make it *behave*. And then you are stuck—behaving, conforming, turning away from your inner being-ness. That is why people who block their feelings and their thoughts, who are afraid to change, are not letting the light out, and they are less healthy, less alive.

It is written in the Scriptures that you should not hide your light under a bushel. Bushels are the problems that we attach ourselves to, that we hang on to. We live in a society that says don't be vulnerable, don't risk; defend yourself from this light that we can shine out. But we need to risk becoming vulnerable to start living. When we shine with our inner light, every cell in our bodies gets the chance to transform. Then we will have insights, greater levels of consciousness, and healthier bodies. For healing means to bring the light forth as it originally was.

You might not realize it, but you are a source of both light and sound waves. Scientists know that light sometimes behaves like waves and sometimes like particles, and they describe light as "wavicles." So you are actually a bunch of wavicles! And you are also sounding out, not just through your voice, but through every particle of your body. Some of you sound like old records—scratchy. Others sound like gorgeous music and are radiant beings. Then, sometimes you are not heard, but you are felt. In fact, all your senses can be so expanded that you can feel, sense, smell, and taste another person. Everyone and every physical object in your environment sends out radiant energy. Some of them radiate short waves, some of them long waves, but the energy is always there.

It is said, "If thine eye could be single, thy whole body would be filled by light." This means that although our bodies are always filled with light, we stagnate and do not activate our energy. We do not allow it to come out as light. Instead, we doubt and judge and divide ourselves from the universe.

While visiting Egypt, I was struck by the symbolism of the eye of Horus. The mythological story is that when the god of the Underworld, Osiris, and Isis brought forth Horus, the uncle of Horus, Set, became jealous of Osiris. He fought Osiris and, as a punishment, he took out one of Horus's eyes. Now Horus had only one eye and could see only one truth. He could not divide any longer. He saw the good in everything in the whole world.

When you shine your light, you shine out everything you are and you touch upon the lives of everything that exists, even beyond this planet Earth. When I listen to the solar music, I can hear the sun and some planets, with their pulsar rays. We, too, are like planets, emitting pulsar rays. Sometimes you meet people and you can feel that they are exciting you, awakening the stagnant forces in you. They do not necessarily have to speak, because they express themselves by their beingness. There is a reason we say silence is golden and speech is silver. You may note that we give silver to people as a laxative.

But imperfections within our bodies break the rhythm of our music. When you are not in rhythm with the continuously transforming energy of the universe, you affect your environment as much as you do when your light is in rhythm. We radiate out those things that are not good for our environment.

"Let there be light and there was light," and it was called good. Yet we have begun to think that opening up to our inner light is bad. It is our lack of understanding of our own inner being. If we look deep into ourselves, we will find that we have the ability to acknowledge our own inner power of light. Shine it on any part of your being that is seemingly not functioning properly, and you will begin to discover your own power of healing, your own path to radiant health.

Our function in life is to expand our consciousness, not by just studying, but by doing and acting. That means letting go of our defenses and opening up to our inner light, which cannot be offended. Shine your light and be active in every part of your being—soul, mind, and body. All the beautiful things you study about body and mind control do not mean a thing unless you put them into practice by being a healthy, self-sufficient individual.

No one wants to be ill, but I say that "I-L-L" stands for "I lack love." Love yourself, because love is the actual activity of the light. When you say, "I love it," you cannot help but feel the excitement move through your body.

In the very high emotional state of love for another person, we can do miracles. A mother can lift a car weighing tons with one hand because she wants to save her child. Can you imagine her suddenly stopping to think about how heavy the car is? If she did, she couldn't lift it an inch. But she doesn't stop to think or doubt. She has total faith in her own ability and inwardly *knows*. Isn't it strange that we require such a tremendous emotional need to bring out that love in our daily life? Can we not bring out the same power of love in every action?

We can. Our inner light is like a laser beam that has the power to heal and free us. How often have you suddenly said, "Now I know—it's like a streak of light that just hit me"? You can't explain it. You just know. And you know that you know, but you don't know how. It is your heart that speaks. It is your own inner light.

I would like to close this book with a meditation on light, its effect on you, and your effect on it. The meditation is called the "rainbow meditation."

Sit, relax, and close your eyes. Take a deep, abdominal breath. Inhale and hold it in. Then release it with a sigh. Now look against your own eyelids as if you were looking into the distance, and imagine that you are standing on a knoll in a gorgeous green meadow looking at a perfect, cloudless, light blue sky. On the horizon there is a fantastic, beautiful, exciting rainbow. Become aware of the rainbow and feel how it touches you. How much are you relating to it and with it? Look over the gorgeous meadow of growth and your horizon where your rainbow is shining on you. You are shining back on the rainbow and feel connected with it. Observe that even though there are many colors, there is still a unity in the multiplicity. It is a whole rainbow, showing its different qualities, its different attributes.

When you gaze at your rainbow, look at the color closest to you—the beautiful, brilliant, vermilion red. Feel it shining on you, warming you, penetrating every part of your being. Red is the life vitality, the life-promoting energy, the energy that activates, the energy that restores and regenerates, that makes stagnant forces become active again. It is stimulating and activating every particle in your body, giving fuel to all those particles that were stagnating. It is the color of the blood streaming through you, the color of your excitement.

Gaze slightly higher, and become aware of the color orange, and allow the golden orange to shine, straight into your heart. Orange is the color of consciousness, combining the red of the body with the yellow of the mind. It is the color of awareness and awakening, the color of the sun, of the heart, the color that harmonizes and restores your rhythm. In the orange of consciousness you are able to express in a perfect way, in a shining way, like the sun, and reflecting like the moon to our fellow man. The orange penetrates every part of your body, gives each cell its own consciousness and its knowledge of its own function. It lets every organ act on its capacity to coordinate and cooperate with all other organs in the body. It has the healing effect of making the body aware of its own consciousness, its knowledge of the universal laws of life continuously transforming.

Go up higher and see the canary yellow, the power of the mind, the direction-giving force, cooling us, giving us insight. Yellow is the intellectual capacity to articulate what we are. Articulation also means to shine out what we are, articulating our potentials, recognizing the omnipotence of God that we are part of, too.

Now see the gorgeous green, the life-preserving color of ecology, the color of seeding, fertilizing, and nurturing, the cooling, naturally healing color of spiritual evolution, the garden of your life. Green combines the yellow of intellect with the blue of volition. The ever-transforming capacities of light within us preserve that life as it was found already within its seed. For within the seed we can find the totality of all that exists, bringing forth orchards of fruit.

Now look up higher to the blue, the color of willpower. See it fade out of its royal blue state of "I will" to the sky blue of "not *my* will, but *thy* will be done." Blue is the color of volition, regulating the expression of your inner knowing. Blue is the color of overcoming your ego and listening to the still, inner voice; it is what makes you know and decide what cools you down, what gives you light.

Now look at the indigo, the forever moving, transforming color, the symbol of transition. Here is the red of vitality, the blue of willpower, and the green of growth, blended and merged together.

Finally, look at the purple, the color of the glory of integration with the universe. See the purple, the lilac, the lavender. The below and the above have become one. We are now all one and regally shining out our total light, integrating every part of our bodies with our whole environment, and expanding this environment throughout the whole universe, as a proof of the multiplicity in unity. We are all that which was in it, an integrated state of consciousness, of physical, mental, and spiritual health or wholeness. You feel the readiness to become transpersonal and to become indeed whole.

Let all these colors now be activated. Shine out as bright, vibrant light, the white light of truth. The truth will set you free. Release this bright white light, the healing, the all encompassing light of your being, and let it shine through the universe. Now, draw the rainbow toward you and blend with it. Feel it penetrating into you and reflect it back at your sky. It has become brighter and brighter as if we all have become like suns in the sky, healing bodies of energy.

Now very slowly, become body-conscious again. Feel and experience the changes that have taken place in your own being and let yourself flow freely with joy and excitement. Take a deep breath. Let it go with a sigh. Take another breath and let it go with a sigh. Now open your eyes. Thank you very, very much for sharing your love with me.